PRESCRIPTIONS FOR HEALTH

Dr Howard Jones

COLLINS

DR HOWARD JONES graduated with a first-class Honours degree in chemistry from University College, Cardiff. The work for his Master's degree, undertaken in collaboration with the Welsh National School of Medicine, was begun in the Physics Department in Cardiff and completed in the Chemistry Department of Imperial College, London.

After a one-year Research Assistantship at the Postgraduate Medical School of London, he worked for his PhD in the King Edward Memorial Hospital in Perth, Western Australia, under the University Department of Biochemistry. This was followed by a further two and a half years' postdoctoral study at McGill Medical School, Montreal, Canada.

For the past fourteen years Dr Howard Jones has been a publishing editor of scientific journals, texts and reference books, specializing in medical chemistry. Although he has written several scientific papers, this is his first full-length book.

He now lives with his wife and son in Dyfed, Wales.

First published in 1986
by William Collins Sons & Co Ltd
London . Glasgow . Sydney
Auckland . Johannesburg

© Howard Jones 1986

British Library Cataloguing in Publication Data

Jones, Howard
   Prescriptions for health.
   1. Nutrition   2. Health
   I. Title
   613.2   RA784

ISBN 0 00 412030 2

Typeset by V & M Graphics Ltd, Aylesbury, Bucks
Printed and bound in Great Britain
by Billing & Sons Ltd, Worcester

PRESCRIPTIONS
FOR HEALTH

CONTENTS

PREFACE

This book is about health – the dietary, physical and environmental aspects of good health, the detrimental factors producing poor health, and suggestions for what to do if we get ill.

Good health is, in fact, a matter of co-ordinating several different factors: correct nutrients, sufficient and appropriate exercise, positive mental attitude, effective relaxation techniques and minimal environmental pollutants. Devotion to any one of these aspects alone will be less effective than it should be if a more important issue for that individual has been overlooked. Individual needs are paramount.

This book is divided into four parts. After an introductory section explaining some of the ideas we'll need to work with, Part 2 puts some nutritional information and dietary recommendations into perspective by balancing opposing extremes with moderation. I have considered each of the principal nutrients in turn and quoted the amounts obtainable from food sources where appropriate.

Vitamins and minerals are discussed in two sections. Part 2 gives a general introduction to the role of these nutrients, and in Part 4 seventeen vitamins and seventeen minerals are considered in detail under the headings of their function in the body, how much we need of each and where we get them from, and finally what happens if we get too much or too little.

The chapter on diet in Part 2 describes the features of ten of the most popular diet schemes, discussing their advantages and disadvantages.

All of this is expressed as simply as possible, emphasizing what is really known about nutrient biochemistry with the minimum of speculation. Explanations are provided of what the body does with its nutrients, and technical biochemical terms are given (*in italics*) to enable interested readers to refer to other books and reviews, including more sophisticated ones if they wish. Nutrition enthusiasts will occasionally come across technical terms they won't have met previously. With the aid of the index, they can look up these terms in the text and find what I hope will be a simple and intelligible explanation.

The subsequent chapters of Part 2 deal in turn with the role of exercise in health, and with energy – where we get it from, what to do with it, and how to balance input with output. This theme is developed, in Chapter 14, 'The Good-health Plan', where dietary and exercise recommendations are pulled together to give schemes which will enable readers to gain, lose, or maintain weight, depending on their individual needs. Part 2 ends with a discussion of two other contributions to health – sex and sleep – with some hints on how to get enough of both.

In Part 3, 'The Body in Disease', we look first at drugs and allergy, of the conventional type as well as food and environmental allergy, and I've mentioned some of the latest techniques of treatment. Then we move on to alternative medicine.

When things go wrong with our health, we have to see a doctor, either of the orthodox school or from one of the alternative practices. There is little I can say which is likely to illuminate people's views of general practitioners or prescription medicine, though some common home remedies are included in the chapter on drugs. With alternative medicine, however, the situation is different.

Practitioners trained in medical schools tend to be, at best, sceptical if not openly contemptuous of alternative medicine. In order to gain what they feel is respectability, alternative therapists try hard to justify their practices in scientific terms, some of which are reasonable, some not. What I have tried to do here is to sort out those aspects of alternative medicine which can be interpreted in rational terms and which perhaps merit further scientific exploration. Those which invoke psychic phenomena belong to the realm of metaphysics and have no place in a book of science. That's not to say, however, that they are not effective in certain cases, even if they cannot be rationally interpreted.

Part 4 is for reference rather than straight-through reading, and includes details of the vitamins and minerals, and a list of books which provide further information on most of the topics described here. I have used many of these texts myself in preparing this book.

I hope that the material, though detailed, is accessible to people who are interested in the care and maintenance of their bodies but who have had no formal scientific training. There should be enough information here to enable anyone to select their own route to health and fitness.

NOTE ABOUT UNITS

In this book it will often be necessary to refer to quantities of the various substances being discussed. In order to deal with quantities of things we must have units.

The tendency in science nowadays, as in everyday life, is to work in the metric system, rather than using Imperial units. The approximate equivalents between Imperial and metric units which are relevant to this book are given below, together with some multiples and sub-multiples of metric units that will need to be used.

Weights (strictly speaking, masses) are measured in kilograms
1 kilogram (kg) = 1,000 grams, which is roughly 2¼ pounds weight
1 gram (g) = 1,000 milligrams (mg) = 1,000,000 micrograms (mcg)
1 ounce is just under 30 grams

Volumes (or, more precisely, capacities) are measured in litres
1 litre (l) = 1,000 millilitres (ml), which is just under 2 pints
1 pint = 20 fluid ounces (UK) or 16 fluid ounces (US) = 568 millilitres or approximately ½ litre

Energy is now measured in joules (J)
1 calorie (cal) is just over 4 joules
   Calories can be a problem, in more ways than one. Books on nutrition generally work in thousands of calories (kilocalories [kcal] or Calories, with a capital C). You will need to check carefully to see which sort is being used in any book you refer to.
1 kilojoule (kJ) = 1,000 joules = 0.24 Calories (or kilocalories) = 240 calories
1 megajoule (MJ) = 1,000 kJ

Percentages expressed in the text are all quoted as weight-for-weight (w/w); that is, 20 per cent of a component in a foodstuff means there are 20 g of the compound in every 100 g (3½ oz) of that food. As the density of water is 1 g per cubic centimetre, 20 per cent of a substance in solution means 20 g in 100 ml of water or 200 g/l.
   Low concentrations, such as those encountered with fluoride in water,

are expressed in parts per million, abbreviated to ppm.

In looking at the weights of ingredients in foods or tablet supplements, you'll need to be careful in interpreting some of the values. Thus, children's fluoride tablets containing 2.2 mg of sodium fluoride have in fact only 1 mg of fluoride (the other 1.2 mg is sodium). Vitamin E tablet supplements often contain chemically prepared dl-tocopherol, a mixture of two different compounds. Only the d- form is active in the body, so the amount of useful vitamin E you get is half the amount of dl-tocopherol specified on the bottle. There are several others like this.

Part 1

INTRODUCTION

1

CELLS AND NUTRIENTS

The improvement in our standard of health this century is due only in small part to the development of sophisticated drugs and expensive surgical hardware. By far the greatest benefits have come from two other sources – the improvements in public health and in nutrition.

In order to stay alive and function adequately the body must have certain nutrients. These are the basic chemicals that make up the structure of the body and which nourish it and provide it with energy.

Some of these essential chemicals are supplied directly to the body in the food that we eat. For others, we must take in the raw materials, the building blocks out of which our bodies can make or *synthesize* the chemicals it needs. All these biochemical maintenance reactions, which are described collectively as *metabolism*, are carried out by cells.

The seven groups of nutrients

The raw materials with which the cells work are supplied by seven groups of compounds. These are the basic nutrients with which we must supply our bodies through our diet. They are: water, proteins, carbohydrates, lipids, vitamins, minerals and fibre. We shall deal with each one of these in turn later on.

How the cells work

Let's look for a moment at the structure of the body. The whole body is made up of *cells*: these are the fundamental biological building blocks. Each cell is surrounded by a wall called a *membrane*. A cell is kept alive by nutrients passing into the cell and waste material moving out through this membrane wall. It's a little like the air bricks in the walls of houses, which let air through into the cavity and allow any moisture trapped in the cavity to get out.

So it is with membranes. They let useful chemicals into the cell and then, when the cell has extracted what it needs, the membrane allows the waste products out. Membranes are also very good at letting in chemicals which the cell wants, but shutting out others which will do the cell harm; or keeping the nutrients in while they let out the waste. The membrane is highly selective about which chemicals it allows to pass through (we say it is *semi-permeable*).

When cells join together in a network they form *tissue*. Cells are the biological units out of which tissues are made. The whole of the solid structure of the body is made up of tissue: skin and bone, nerves and muscles are all tissues. When two or more tissues are joined together with a specific biological function, that collection of tissues is called an *organ*: the heart and brain, lungs and kidneys are all organs.

All the organs and tissues are therefore made up of cells. We know that the brain, the liver, and the skin, say, all look very different. Apart from being different shapes and sizes, the brain is pink-grey and spongy, the liver is brownish-red, smooth and compact, while the skin is pinkish-white, covered with holes (*pores*), and is built up in layers which tend to peel off if we stay out too long in the sun.

The individual cells that make up the various tissues and organs reflect this difference in external appearance, and they themselves differ considerably in their shape, size, and detailed structure. They also differ in the type and amount of large organic molecules they contain. But irrespective of the function of a cell, the nature and proportion of the smaller inorganic components is remarkably similar from one cell to another.

The body's chemicals

We shall need to talk quite a lot about organic and inorganic compounds in our bodies. *Organic compounds* are those which make up the substance of living things. They all contain carbon, together with the elements oxygen and hydrogen. They also often contain nitrogen, sulphur and phosphorus, and occasionally there are metal atoms like iron or cobalt present. Proteins, carbohydrates and lipids are all organic substances.

Inorganic compounds are those made up from the rest of the ninety or so elements, excluding carbon. Water, salt and silica are examples of inorganic compounds. For the most part, inorganic elements travel around the body either as single atoms or in groups of atoms called *radicals* and carrying a positive or negative charge. These charged atoms or radicals are called *ions*.

The inorganic ions which are found in the greatest concentration inside the cell (in *intracellular fluid*) are potassium and the phosphate radical, with very much smaller amounts of magnesium and the sulphate radical. Outside the cell (in the *extracellular fluid*) the ions sodium and chloride dominate. This applies no matter what the function of the tissue. It is to nourish the cells of these tissues that we eat, drink, exercise, and cultivate our minds. This provides the chemical nutrients and the physical stimulation that tissues need for continued health.

Our bodies are made up almost completely of the lighter elements,

3

which have smaller atoms. This is because these elements are more abundant and their atoms are more mobile; they can also be packed more easily than larger atoms into chemical assemblages called *molecules* without leaving spaces between the atoms.

There is an interesting comparison we can make in relation to the elements in organic and inorganic compounds. Organic compounds have been defined as those which contain carbon. They also all contain hydrogen. Why should this be so? It is because hydrogen atoms are just the right size to pack around a carbon atom without leaving any large gaps between them. The arrangement is so stable that the carbons and hydrogens often form long chains, as in the fatty acids (see Chapter 6); or rings, as in vitamin B12 (see Chapter 26).

In the inorganic world of the rocks there is another atom, similar to carbon in some ways, which forms the basic skeleton of many geological minerals. This is the element silicon that we now hear so much about in relation to microcomputers. Silicon can also form chains and rings, just like carbon, but this time it isn't hydrogen atoms which join up with the silicon. These would be too small and there would be a lot of space between them. The space-filling atom now is oxygen. Silicon and oxygen form extended structures (*silicates*) in geological minerals in a way that is comparable to carbon and hydrogen in organic materials.

This idea of packing atoms together to fill up the available space is fundamental to the stability of the structures of both organic and inorganic compounds. As we shall see, the ability of proteins to form stable long chains is the reason why some of them function as enzymes to control our body's chemistry (see Chapter 10).

How the nutrients are used

There are three basic ways that nutrients are put to use by cells:

1   To build and repair tissue.
2   To provide energy.
3   To eliminate toxins, excess raw materials from food, and unwanted products from the body's chemical reactions.

1   The substance of most of the solid tissues of our body is protein. The same is true for animals. Chapter 4 will explain how the body breaks down protein foods and reassembles the components to provide other proteins we require for structural tissue or enzymes.

The one major tissue of the body which is not predominantly protein is bone. Only one-third of bone is organic matter, the other two-thirds being inorganic, mostly calcium carbonate and calcium phosphate.

2   Energy in the body is derived mainly from carbohydrates and lipids

(which each contribute some 45 per cent of the total) and from proteins (the remaining 10 per cent).

Energy is used for conscious movement of our limbs, for driving the heart and lungs, for producing contractions of the muscle walls of the stomach and intestines to enable us to digest our food, and to carry out chemical reactions in the body. Energy sources and uses are discussed in more detail in Chapter 13.

3 Elimination of waste from the body occurs through three routes. Our skin has tiny pores through which we lose water and salts in the form of sweat. We need water to flush soluble salts and *urea* (derived from the nitrogen content of proteins) through the kidneys and out of the body as urine. Solids are processed by the gut – stomach and intestines – and require roughage or fibre to assist the passage of waste material as faeces (see also Chapter 9 and pages 52–54).

Most of the liquid we excrete passes out of the body as sweat or urine. Only some 100 to 200 ml of liquid passes each day through the rectum in normal conditions. In diarrhoea the amount is considerably greater, sometimes enough to produce dehydration.

The body takes just what it needs from dietary nutrients and eliminates the excess and waste through one of the above three routes. This state of dynamic equilibrium between nutrients and tissues is called *homeostasis*.

Summary: how we use nutrients from food

The seven groups of raw materials we require for health are used by the body mainly as follows:

1 **Water:** for circulation of nutrients, lubrication of joints and organs, and elimination of waste.
2 **Proteins:** to make structural tissue, enzymes to control the body's biochemical reactions, and antibodies to fight infection.
3 **Carbohydrates:** for energy.
4 **Lipids:** for energy, and to assist in the biochemical processing of food.
5 **Vitamins:** diverse uses, some as yet unknown, but generally involved in biochemical reaction control.
6 **Minerals:** various uses, but, like vitamins, generally involved in biochemical reaction control.
7 **Fibre:** for elimination of toxins and waste by slowing the process of mastication (chewing), and by dispersing or bulking out the food mass, helping in the absorption of nutrients.

In addition, there are two sets of compounds – enzymes and hormones – which are used in reaction control and which are manufactured in the body (see Chapter 10).

This simplification gives a broad overview of how we use the food we eat. We shall look at each type of nutrient in more detail in Parts 2 and 4.

2

THE AVERAGE PERSON

Individuality

One of the fundamental principles that we need to appreciate at the outset on the road to improved health and fitness is that every person is different. This may seem to be self-evident, yet so many books on diet or exercise carry with them, in their recommendations, the implication that what is prescribed is suitable for everyone. I believe that not enough attention is paid to individual requirements.

We meet this even in the standards that are set officially for intake of the various nutrients. Most textbooks of conventional nutrition quote Recommended Daily Allowances (RDA values) for dietary components, and we need to get these into perspective.

The UK RDA value for vitamin C, for example, is 30 mg. This is claimed to be adequate for all normal, healthy individuals. But is this amount enough just to protect against scurvy (the vitamin C deficiency disease), or will it also give increased immunity from colds and respiratory tract infections, or help prevent cancer developing in twenty years' time, if indeed vitamin C does any of these things as some people claim?

Nobel Prizewinner Linus Pauling has long advocated a daily intake of several grams of vitamin C. Which of these recommended values is correct? Perhaps the truth lies somewhere between the two.

What is certain is that neither 30 mg nor 5 g of vitamin C daily is right for everyone. There are many people for whom daily vitamin or mineral supplements are almost certainly a waste of money. On the other hand, there are others who definitely do benefit from increased – sometimes greatly increased – daily doses of vitamins.

Another factor which highlights the confusion about how much of each vitamin we really need is the considerable difference in recommended intake values from one country to another. Thus, although the UK recommended value for vitamin C intake is only 30 mg, in the US it is 60 mg and in the USSR it is 120 mg. Is this discrepancy due to different metabolism of typical individuals in the population, or to different environmental factors, or simply to different opinions? This wide divergence in recommended values is not found with all nutrients, but it does indicate that for some at least, especially vitamin C, there is a considerable amount of latitude in optimal daily intake. The vitamin C controversy is discussed in more detail in Chapter 26.

One further point should be mentioned here, though we shall meet it again in various sections later: this is the question of quantity of nutrient available. The nutrient in a food source may be locked in chemically in such a way that we cannot extract it; or it may be partially destroyed by cooking or processing; or it may be available to one person but not to another with a different metabolism.

The RDA values given for daily intake of all nutrients are *average* values – the significance of these will be discussed in a moment. If you are particularly slim or overweight, energetic or lethargic, or if you have a high daily intake of cigarettes or alcohol or other drugs, your requirements for nutrients will be different – usually higher, occasionally lower.

Similarly, conventional pharmaceuticals are dispensed in standard dosages. What may be optimal for one person may have little effect on another and be too strong for a third.

So it is important really to believe in the statement that you are an individual. You can take advice from medical practitioners, orthodox or alternative, consult your diet cookbook, work your way through the Jane Fonda exercise tape; but in the end, it's *your* body and only you can decide what to do with it – whether the prescribed drugs are too strong for you or are having distressing side effects, whether something in that delicious and nutritious health recipe brings you out in a rash, or whether that hamstring stretch is really more than you can cope with.

Averages and ranges

There is one other thing we need to consider about averages, and that is the *range* to which they apply.

Suppose we have a controlled study to see how much of a certain nutrient is used up in a given period of time. The lowest value of nutrient used is 45 mg and the highest value is 55 mg. The range in this case (the difference between the lowest and the highest figures) is 10 mg. Let us assume the average of the experimental values turns out to be 50 mg. This means the average value is much higher than the range.

Suppose instead that the experiments had yielded values of nutrient used which varied from 20 mg to 80 mg, a range of 60 mg; and let's suppose the average is once again 50 mg. This time the average is smaller than the range.

The underlying principle here is this: if the range of values is small in comparison with the average, then the average value is significant. If, however, the range is large compared with the average, then your own requirements of that nutrient may be very different from the RDA value. The important point to stress is that the quoted average values of nutrients which are required by different individuals and those which are found in various foods are often associated with quite considerable ranges, which makes the published average figures at best of dubious value and at times quite meaningless.

The problem we face is that ranges are rarely ever quoted along with the tables giving RDA values in standard textbooks, so we have no idea of their significance. The ranges will often be given in the original research papers, but these are not accessible to a general readership. Once again, therefore, you must make up your own mind as to what you need, and use the published figures only as a guide. The following chapters will give you tips on how to make these decisions.

Part 2

THE HEALTHY BODY

3
WATER

Although we can live for a month or more without food, we can survive for only a few days without water. It is definitely an essential nutrient.

Distribution

Water is a part of every cell and tissue of our body. It occurs either inside the cells (*intracellular fluid*, 55 per cent) or outside (*extracellular fluid*, 45 per cent). The fluid outside the cells includes such things as the light, straw-coloured liquid (*plasma*) which remains when we take the cells away from blood. The backup liquid circulating system (*lymph*) that we have in the body for fighting infections is largely water; so is the fluid (*cerebrospinal fluid*) that surrounds the brain in the skull and the spinal cord in the backbone, and which acts as a shock absorber and medium for transport of nutrients.

The water content of our tissues shows a wide variation: our blood is 90 per cent water, but fatty (*adipose*) tissue is only 20 per cent water. Water occurs in much smaller quantities between the organs and within the joints (*synovial fluid*) to act as a lubricant.

The proportion of water in our bodies decreases with age. Almost three-quarters (75 per cent) of the weight of a newborn baby is water, while in a sixty-year-old that proportion has dropped to about half (50 per cent). This is one of the factors contributing to wrinkling of the skin in old age – loss of water content of both the skin itself and the underlying tissue bulk.

Intake

We take in about 3 l (5 pints) of water each day, which corresponds to a weight of water of 3 kg (6½ lb). Half of this is in the form of drinks (tea, coffee, milk, beer, etc., as well as water itself). Another litre (1¾ pints) is in our solid food, and the remainder is formed inside the body by the burning (*combustion*) of sugars and other energy-producing compounds. Foods like melon, celery, broccoli and lettuce are more than 90 per cent water. Only obviously dried foods, like cream crackers, or fatty foods such as butter and some cheeses have less than a 20 per cent water content.

Water has no energy value and therefore, by itself, is in no way fattening. The amount of water you drink will not affect your overall weight, for any excess will be excreted over the following few hours. Only if you eat too much fat and carbohydrate, or take too little exercise, will the water in your diet contribute to weight gain. You cannot prevent weight gain by not drinking water since you will get ample from the food you eat to shore up the fatty tissue. Only when the fatty tissue which holds the water is broken down will there be weight loss. It is the sugar and milk in tea and coffee that puts on weight, not the water. The more water you drink the better, in order to flush waste products through the kidneys.

Output

Water is one of the media of excretion from the body in the form of sweat and urine. The pores of the skin excrete a watery solution containing mainly dissolved sodium chloride (salt), together with smaller amounts of other mineral salts and urea. The urea comes mainly from the nitrogen of proteins.

Apart from its function in excretion, one role of sweat is to regulate the body temperature. When we are hot, we perspire more and the evaporation of the water cools us down. (This is what the physicists call the Joule-Kelvin effect. We have to do work to tear liquid molecules apart and convert them to gas. The energy required to do this work is taken as heat from the body.) The degree of sweating is under the control of a lower portion of the brain (the *hypothalamus*), which is also involved in hormone secretion.

Even at a comfortable room (*ambient*) temperature of 24°C (75°F) we lose something like 600 to 800 ml (1 to 1½ pints) of water through sweating each day. During strenuous exertion we can lose up to 2 l (3½ pints) an hour through perspiration, but on an average day's activity we would reckon to lose about 1 l (1¾ pints) through sweating.

On a normal diet with minimal activity we excrete about 1.5 l (2½ pints) of water each day through urine, and the remaining 0.5 l (¾ pint) (to take us up to the average day's intake) is exhaled through the lungs. That quantity of urine contains about 30 g of urea and smaller quantities of salts, mainly sodium chloride, phosphate, and sulphate. To balance this salt loss we need about 1.5 g of sodium, or 3 g of common salt, each day in our diet.

Thus, we need to take in more water each day, both directly as liquid and indirectly in our food, than any other single nutrient.

Chlorination and fluoridation

Chlorine is added to drinking water supplies to kill (oxidize) harmful bacteria. A trace of the chlorine will stay as the gas, dissolved in water, and it is this that sometimes determines the taste and may contribute to hypersensitivity reactions in some people.

Most of the chlorine reacts with water to form hydrochloric acid (a normal constituent of gastric juice), together with an unstable, oxygenated form of hydrochloric acid (*hypochlorous acid*). It is this unstable form that gives up its oxygen to kill bacteria. When it does so, it too forms harmless hydrochloric acid. Apart from its effect on the taste of drinking water, chlorination generally does no harm to our bodies, as far as we know.

Some water supplies in Britain and the US are already fluoridated to a concentration of about one part per million (1 ppm) to help prevent dental decay (*caries*). Fluoridation is effected by adding sodium fluoride to the water. In some districts, water is fluoridated naturally, mostly by dissolving small quantities of calcium fluoride from minerals (*fluorspar* and *apatite*) in the rocks.

In the solid state, sodium fluoride and calcium fluoride are very different substances. Sodium fluoride is more toxic only because it is considerably more soluble than calcium fluoride. This leads to the statement sometimes encountered that sodium fluoride is less stable than calcium fluoride.

Once the appropriate solids are dissolved in water at an identical small concentration there is absolutely no difference between fluoride derived from mineral sources and that which is added artificially to the water, despite the claims of environmental protection groups to the contrary. In dilute solution, the metal parts and the fluoride part of these compounds have a more or less independent existence.

One disadvantage cited against fluoridation is that it increases our sodium intake and this is now considered undesirable. However, the amount is so slight as to be negligible in relation to the amount already in our bodies and taken in our food. You will get more sodium from one crisp or one salted peanut than from half a litre (¾ pint) of fluoridated water.

At high concentrations fluoride is undoubtedly a poison. It forms relatively strong chemical links (*hydrogen bonds*) with amides in the proteins in our bodies and may thus disrupt the protein or at least interfere with its normal biological action. Whether or not this is the source of its toxicity is not known.

At the concentration encountered in deliberately fluoridated water (1 ppm or 1 mg/litre) we are taking in about 1.5 mg per day, which is certainly not toxic and is beneficial in strengthening bones and teeth. It is possible to get up to 10 mg per day from naturally fluoridated water in some districts (at 6 ppm), though natural concentrations are usually much less than this. The fluoride question is discussed in full on pages 184–87.

Mineral water

This is natural water containing a higher than average quantity of dissolved mineral salts. It may also be made sparkling by having carbon dioxide dissolved into it artificially.

The main metals found in mineral waters are calcium and magnesium, both natural constituents of the body. There is often about five times as much sodium as potassium, but the amounts are still small. Someone who drinks only mineral water (1.5 l or 2½ pints each day) will get about 150 mg of calcium and up to 15 mg of sodium daily from this source.

The amount of fluoride in mineral water is only about one-tenth of that in artificially fluoridated water (total intake is about 0.2 mg or 200 mcg fluoride in 1.5 l). The other non-metallic elements appear mainly as chlorides and sulphates, both natural components of our bodies.

Table 1   Typical analyses of mineral water. All ion concentrations are in milligrams per litre

Ashbourne Water from Derbyshire, England		Evian Water from France	
calcium	102	calcium	78
magnesium	24	magnesium	24
sodium	10	sodium	5
potassium	1.6	potassium	1
lithium	0.08	bicarbonate	357
iron	0.1	fluoride	0.12
fluoride	0.15	chloride	2.2
chloride	30	sulphate	10
sulphate	60	nitrate	3.8
nitrate/nitrite	trace		
carbon dioxide	3 vols per vol. of water		

Water purity

One advantage of spring water over tap water is its low nitrate content. Nitrate levels in drinking water are allowed up to 100 mg/litre in Britain. With the nitrate ingested from tinned and packaged meats, this represents a disturbingly large total daily intake of a chemical high on the list of suspects as causing stomach cancer. The high nitrate level in ground water in the UK is due to that leached out of the soil from extensive use of artificial fertilizers. As there is no control on the application of nitrate fertilizers, the likelihood is that drinking water levels will get even higher in the future.

The problem is compounded in several parts of Europe and the US by the widespread occurrence of acid rain. Rain falls as dilute sulphuric and nitric acids in some areas after it has dissolved gaseous oxides from the air. The sulphate is no problem, but the nitrate adds to that derived from fertilizers. The main hazard with acid rain, however, is the acidity itself, which leaches essential minerals out of the soil and dissolves metals out of water pipes (quite apart from causing extensive damage to vegetation). The issue is discussed further on page 177.

The European Economic Community (EEC) has established desirable levels of nitrate content in drinking water and of noxious emissions likely to cause acid rain, but so far the UK has not embraced these recommendations for Britain.

It is a mistake to believe that mineral water is *necessarily* more pure than tap water. Mineral water is, after all, only bottled natural spring or ground water, perhaps with a little fizz added. Depending on its source, the water may not be completely free from either chemical or bacteriological contamination. When it is sold in soft, plastic containers, as it is in many supermarkets, it may dissolve small quantities of chemicals from the plastic – minute amounts maybe, but apparently enough to cause allergic reactions in susceptible individuals. So there are no guarantees, even with mineral water.

Drinking only distilled water is not a practicable solution either. A family of four would need about 6 to 8 l (10½ to 14 pints) distilled every day. Also, the taste of distilled water is flat and uninteresting since all the beneficial minerals, such as calcium (which is believed to provide some protection against heart disease), have been removed in the distillation process. A still is quite expensive to buy and to run, and excise officials are likely to develop an increased interest in the family since it can also be used for other less innocuous preparations!

Unless you know the tap water in your area could be contaminated or it has a revolting taste, mineral and distilled waters are expensive, unnecessary and, in some cases, actually disadvantageous alternatives for most of us.

4
PROTEINS

The word 'protein' is derived from the Greek word *protos*, meaning 'first'. These compounds were given their name by the Dutch chemist Gerard Mulder in 1838, because he believed that they were the most important constituents of all living things. Actually, for plants, carbohydrates fill the role that proteins perform in animals.

Distribution

Only water is more abundant as a constituent of the human body. The protein of which we are composed is distributed 35 per cent in our muscles, 20 per cent in bones and cartilage, 10 per cent in skin, and the other 35 per cent in all our organs and body fluids. Urine and bile are the only body fluids which do not usually contain proteins.

What are proteins?

Proteins, carbohydrates and lipids are all made up of carbon, hydrogen and oxygen. Phosphorus and sulphur may be present too, but proteins are unique in always possessing nitrogen in their structure, and it is this nitrogen which is turned into urea.

All proteins are *polymers*; this means they are made up of smaller chemical building blocks joined end-to-end. In the proteins the basic building units are called *amino acids*.

There are about twenty different common amino acids which, in various permutations, make up all the proteins of the animal world: hair, nails, skin, brain tissue, muscle, enzymes; the wool and feathers of animals; and many other variations.

The body can synthesize most of the amino acids from simpler chemical units. There are a few amino acids, however, which must be eaten as such in our food because the body cannot make them. These are called *essential amino acids*, a somewhat unfortunate name perhaps since all twenty amino acids are essential to good health. It is just that we can make the rest for ourselves, provided we have the necessary chemical ingredients (*precursors*) in our bodies.

Authorities differ on just how many of the amino acids should be regarded as essential; some give eight, some as many as ten. These are listed for reference in Table 2.

15

Table 2   The essential and most common 'non-essential' amino acids

Essential	Non-essential
arginine	alanine
histidine	asparagine
isoleucine	aspartate
leucine	cysteine
lysine	glutamate
methionine	glutamine
phenylalanine	glycine
threonine	hydroxyproline
tryptophan	proline
valine	serine
	tyrosine

Notes

1   There is some debate as to whether arginine and histidine should be regarded as essential amino acids. They are manufactured by the body, but not in sufficient quantities for our needs.

2   Some tables list cystine instead of cysteine. Cystine consists of two cysteine molecules joined together (and oxidized by the removal of hydrogen).

3   Asparagine and glutamine are amino forms of aspartate and glutamate respectively, and are not always listed separately.

4   Hydroxyproline is formed in the body by adding oxygen to proline. This is another amino acid not always listed if proline is included.

Proteins are described as *simple* if they are made up only of amino acids, and *compound* or *conjugated* if they are made up of a protein bound to some other type of molecule. The keratin of hair and nails is a simple protein. Haemoglobin in blood is a conjugated protein in which the simple protein, globin, is wound round an iron-containing molecule called haem. In haemoglobin the globin part 'breathes' in and out as it captures or releases oxygen for use by the tissues, the oxygen sitting on the haem part of the molecule.

Another way of describing proteins is on the basis of the shapes of the molecules, which in turn depend on their composition. There are *globular proteins*, which roll up into a ball (like enzymes, antibodies, and haemoglobin), and there are *fibrous proteins*, which look like the strands of a fine cable coiled around each other (like keratin in hair and nails, and myosin in muscle).

Proteins in food

The principal dietary sources of proteins are meat, poultry, fish, eggs, milk and other dairy products, nuts and legumes, with smaller amounts in cereals.

Because Man is a part of the animal kingdom, the proteins derived from animal sources supply the range of amino acids we need more completely than vegetable sources. Eggs are one of the most completely nutritious foods of all.

Nevertheless, by choosing carefully a balanced intake of alternative protein sources, vegetarians and vegans are perfectly able to achieve good health without recourse to animal protein. The main problems arise not with the proteins themselves but with the minor constituents like vitamins and minerals.

The values quoted for minimum or recommended amounts of daily protein intake vary from one source to another, as can be seen below. They are, in any case, somewhat arbitrary and should be taken only as a guide.

The US Federal Register (1973) RDA value is 65 g for poor-quality protein and 45 g for high-quality protein (from foods such as those listed above). The Food and Agriculture Organization (FAO)/WHO (1972) recommended values are 37 g for adult men and 29 g for adult women. The British DHSS (1969) values are a minimum of 45 g and a recommended 60 to 90 g for men (depending on their degree of activity), and the corresponding values for women are 38 g minimum and 48 to 68 g recommended.

I have quoted these values so that you can see something of the degree of variation. If you find all these numbers confusing, let's take 40 g as a working figure for the minimum daily protein intake for an adult man or woman who is reasonably active. If you think you are highly active, add half as much again (work to 60 g). If you are a man doing strenuous manual labouring, work to double the minimum value (80 g) daily. You will not be significantly adrift.

Some steroids, such as cortisol, which is used to treat arthritis, increase the breakdown of proteins; so a diet with higher protein content is also recommended to accompany steroid therapy.

Let's see now what 40 g of protein means in terms of the food we eat. This is equivalent to about 125 g (4½ oz) of lean (fat-trimmed) beef steak or (boneless) chicken breast, 140 g (5 oz) of tuna steak, 155 g (5½ oz) of peanuts, or 200 g (7 oz) of tinned salmon or haddock fillet in breadcrumbs.

One large egg, whether boiled, poached, scrambled or fried (it makes little difference to the amount of protein content), contains about the same amount of protein as a large avocado pear – 5 to 6 g. There are about 21 g of protein in 600 ml (1 pint) of milk, whether or not it is skimmed. Full-fat cheese contains 7 g of protein per 30 g (1 oz) (25 per cent protein, w/w), while cottage cheese has only half as much: a 115 g (4 oz) tub (the usual individual portion) will give 16 g of protein.

To get your daily requirement of protein from cereal alone, you would have to eat about five moderate bowls of a high-protein variety (like Kellogg's Special K) to get 30 g (with another 10 g from 300 ml or ½ pint of milk). Kellogg's Special K is as high as 20 per cent protein, but most cereals contain only 7 to 10 per cent. This information is summarized in Figure 1.

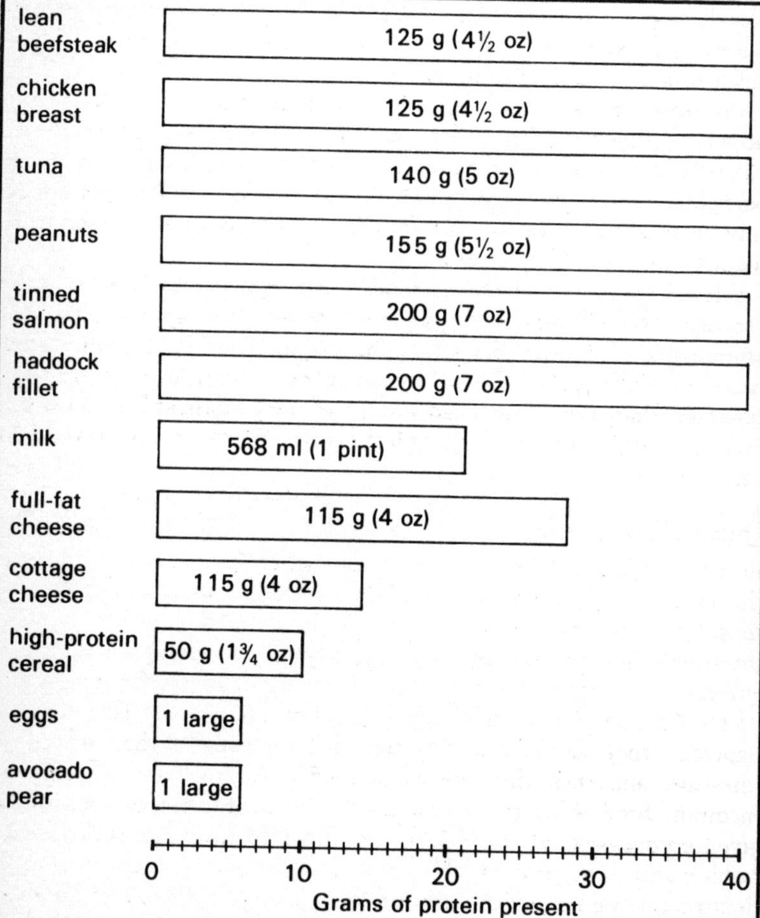

lean beefsteak	125 g (4½ oz)
chicken breast	125 g (4½ oz)
tuna	140 g (5 oz)
peanuts	155 g (5½ oz)
tinned salmon	200 g (7 oz)
haddock fillet	200 g (7 oz)
milk	568 ml (1 pint)
full-fat cheese	115 g (4 oz)
cottage cheese	115 g (4 oz)
high-protein cereal	50 g (1¾ oz)
eggs	1 large
avocado pear	1 large

0   10   20   30   40

Grams of protein present

Figure 1   The protein content (in grams) of some common foods

This will give you a good idea of how much of the high-protein foods you should aim to eat each day. Rather than getting all your protein from one source, it is better to mix your foods, having, say, cereal and milk for breakfast, with an occasional egg; lean meat, fish, or poultry with fresh vegetables at lunch time; and a salad with cheese, prawns, tuna or nuts at tea time. You could rotate just these foods alone, with variations in the specific ingredients, and have an excellent, nutritional, interesting diet every day for a month without ever having the same meal twice.

Applying this variety principle, we could eat a *few* peanuts as an appetizer, or have a *small* glass of milk with a meat or fish meal, or finish with a *small* portion of cheese to enhance the amino acid pool in the blood. Also, protein (or alcohol) before a meal stimulates the digestive juices; so the practice of having a drink with a few peanuts before a meal has a sound physiological basis.

As amino acids are not stored to any great extent in the body, it is important that each day, and preferably each meal if possible, we get as balanced a protein intake as we can. Eating a large amount of one particular protein at a meal, followed by a different protein at a meal four to six hours later will not necessarily provide all the amino acids required for body protein synthesis.

All of the foods listed above contain all of the essential amino acids, to varying degrees. Some foods may be relatively low in one particular amino acid; for example, corn (maize), polished rice, white flour, coconuts and pecans are low in tryptophan. It is reassuring to know, however, that even white bread and white rice contain at least a little of every essential amino acid, though the quantity of some of them is very small.

Digestion of proteins

Proteins are digested both in the stomach and in the intestines. Pepsin is the main protein-breaking (*proteolytic*) enzyme in the stomach; but most of the protein digestion (*lysis* and *absorption*) is carried out by the intestinal enzymes (*trypsin, chymotrypsin* and *carboxypeptidase*). These enzymes come from the pancreas and are activated by the intestine.

This is an ingenious piece of biology. If the enzymes were active in the pancreas, they would attack it. Instead, they are shipped off to the intestine, and then they are activated so that they attack only the incoming food. Also, the gut has a specially lined wall (coated with the *glycoprotein, mucin*) to resist attack either by the acidic gastric juice (which contains hydrochloric acid) or by enzymes. If this lining breaks down, acid and enzymes get through to the wall itself and a peptic ulcer may be formed (gastric in the stomach; duodenal in the intestine).

The body takes in the protein in food; then enzymes chop up each protein, first into smaller fragments (*polypeptides*), and eventually into individual amino acids which circulate in the blood. Other enzymes reassemble the constituent amino acids in the order required for the specific body protein.

This amino acid pool is needed throughout life, either to build new tissue or replenish that which exists already; but the reserve requirement decreases with age as the rate of the body's biochemical reactions (*metabolism*) slows down.

The starting point in the body for the manufacture of most of the 'non-essential' amino acids is glutamate. In fact, the levels of both glutamate and aspartate found in the blood are low, since they are converted largely into alanine. It is believed that glutamate and aspartate take metal ions like calcium and magnesium out of circulation (by *chelation*). Consequently, glutamate is one amino acid the body cannot tolerate in large quantities, such as may be found in tinned soups and in certain Chinese food. The headache, nausea, palpitations and bloated feeling sometimes experienced after eating such food with a high concentration of monosodium glutamate are due to an excess of glutamate in the intestine – more than the body can cope with. For this reason its use is banned in baby foods. A small quantity of monosodium glutamate, which is widely used as a food additive to enhance flavour, is however quite harmless. Both the sodium and glutamate are natural constituents of the body.

The sulphur-containing amino acids, cysteine and methionine, are also toxic if they are present at too high a concentration; but the body has in-built mechanisms to overcome this problem.

During the processes of digestion, amino acids are converted into a whole range of different compounds. Serine is converted to compounds (*phospholipids*) which form an integral part of cell membranes. Glycine forms haem, which is used in oxygen-carrying haemoglobin in the blood and which is a component of the energy storage and transfer systems (in *cytochrome*).

Phenylalanine is converted into tyrosine. If the body does not have the ability to carry this out, the phenylalanine reaches toxic levels in the blood and, if not checked, would ultimately lead to mental retardation. This condition can be tested for by the presence of phenylalanine and phenylketone in the urine – it is known as *phenylketonuria*. Such a test is now carried out routinely on newborn babies.

Tyrosine, in turn, is converted into the body pigment melanin, which gives us a sun-tan. It is tyrosine which also provides the major amino acid starting point for generating the iodine-containing thyroid hormone (*l-thyroxine*) and for the hormones of the adrenal gland (*catecholamines: adrenaline* and *noradrenaline*).

Proteins and energy

Most of the energy needs of the body are provided by carbohydrates and lipids. Only some 10 per cent of this energy comes from amino acids in normal conditions. If, however, the energy supply from normal routes is insufficient – as in people who are deliberately cutting down on fats and carbohydrates as part of a slimming diet – the body may turn to valuable amino acids instead as an energy source. The amino acids may be burned for immediate energy, or they may be converted into carbohydrates and lipids and stored for energy required later.

When amino acids are burned, they are converted into carbon dioxide and water, and the nitrogen is turned into urea, which is excreted by the kidneys. A high-protein diet produces a high level of urea excretion.

Proteins and fasting

If someone goes on a fasting diet, whether from choice or necessity, it is important that protein intake is increased gradually when the fast is over (see page 51). The enzymes which break down amino acids increase during starvation to provide energy for survival from body proteins. High protein intake at this point produces indigestion, at best, or in extreme cases may lead to death from ammonia poisoning.

After fasting, the diet should contain high carbohydrate and low protein for a few days, until the level of amino-acid-burning enzymes is lowered. Then the protein should be increased gradually.

A low-protein diet over an extended period of time can also produce a fatty liver, a condition which is difficult to reverse. This arises because there are insufficient protein carriers to take fat out of the liver to other parts of the body where the fat can be burned to satisfy the body's energy requirement.

5
CARBOHYDRATES

CARBOHYDRATE CHEMISTRY

Carbohydrates are so called because they all contain carbon, hydrogen and oxygen, and the latter two types of atoms are in the same ratio as they occur in water, namely two to one. Carbohydrates do not contain any water as such, despite their name.

What are carbohydrates?

We obtain carbohydrates in our diet from potatoes, cereals, fruit and vegetables, bread and cakes, puddings and sweets.

Digestible carbohydrates are of two types: starches and sugars. We can tell the difference between these by their taste – sugars are sweet, starches are not. There is also a chemical difference.

Starches: these belong to the group of chemicals called polymers. Like the proteins, starches are made up by repeating chemical building blocks over and over. With proteins there are about twenty different units that can be joined together – the amino acids. With starches the picture is much simpler: there is only one type of building block, and that is glucose. The glucose units are joined up end-to-end or side-to-side, in an indefinitely long chain (to form a *polysaccharide*).

Starch is a mixture of two different substances, both polymers. In one of these the glucose building blocks are joined in a straight chain; in the other the glucose units form a branched chain. Starch obtained from different plants has different amounts of these two compounds. Because of the amount of the branched polymer that is present, starch is only sparingly soluble in water.

Most of the carbohydrate in potatoes is starch, which makes up about 20 per cent of their weight when peeled. Cereals like wheat and corn contain up to 70 per cent starch, and even dried peas and beans have up to 40 per cent of their dry weight taken up by starch. Starch is the food reserve of the plant – it fulfils the same role in the plant as glycogen does in our bodies.

Sugars: these are carbohydrates made up of just one or two chemical units (called *monosaccharides* and *disaccharides* respectively). They are not polymers.

There are only three types of double-unit sugars in food: maltose, lactose, and sucrose.

Maltose is found, as the name suggests, in malt, which is prepared by the fermenting of grains, particularly barley. Maltose is made up of two glucose units joined together and is a relatively small component of the diet.

Lactose is also a minor dietary constituent and is found only in milk. In its chemical structure it has a glucose molecule joined to a different type of building unit, galactose.

The third double-unit sugar is by far the most common and most important in the diet: this is *sucrose*, which is composed chemically of a glucose unit joined to a third type of building unit, fructose. Sucrose is the end-product of crystallization of the juice of sugar cane or sugar beet. The sugars prepared in this way, whether brown or white, are 98 to 99 per cent pure sucrose.

White, granulated sugar has been refined and in the process has lost virtually all of its micronutrients. Demerara sugar, named after the district of Guyana where it was first prepared, Muscovado or Barbados sugar and all other brown sugars may have been refined, or may not – we have to look at the packaging to find out. Packets of unrefined sugar should always have their country of origin printed on them, most usually Guyana, Barbados or Mauritius. They may, in addition, have a list of the micronutrient minerals which they contain, together with their concentrations. Packets of refined sugar, on the other hand, will show no such country of origin as they are refined in the country where they are consumed. In addition, they may have a list of the colourings and flavourings used so that it will be obvious that the sugar is no longer in its natural state. Refined brown sugar is no better nutritionally than white, and also has the disadvantage of containing additives.

The colour of brown sugars, natural or refined, is due to molasses or caramel. Molasses is the uncrystallizable syrup which remains at the end of the crystallization process in refining. As well as imparting colour, the presence of molasses gives brown sugar a distinctive flavour and a moist, sticky appearance.

Caramel or burnt sugar is widely used as a dark brown colouring (E150) for many foods apart from sugar (like brown biscuits, sweet pickle, soy sauce or breakfast cereals). If it has been prepared simply by heating, it is less likely to cause hypersensitivity problems than if it has been prepared from sugar by the addition of chemicals, which is often the case.

There is a tendency for some health food devotees to regard sugar almost as a poison. In fact, it is one of the purest foods and it supplies us with essential energy. As we shall see, however, there are reasons why we should moderate our intake: most of us probably eat far too much sugar, but there is certainly no need to avoid it altogether. If you want to use sugar in its most natural form, complete with minerals, you need to use raw, brown sugar, without adulterated caramel, prepared in its country of origin.

If you want to minimize your sugar intake you need to be on the alert for otherwise health-giving and natural foods which have been already sweetened before packaging. Tins of soup or baked beans, breakfast cereals (especially muesli) and flavoured yoghurts frequently have sugar added. Baked beans, for example, usually contain about 4 per cent added sugar. Many vitamin pills are also coated with sugar (and synthetic dyes!).

In the UK the usual practice now is to list ingredients in decreasing order of quantity present: sugar is often at the top of the list after the main component. In the US manufacturers are required to list specific amounts of ingredients, and this practice is increasing in the UK. As you get into the habit of reading labels you will soon be aware that different brands of the same product differ significantly in content, so you can select on the basis of this and the taste.

We have seen that there are just three types of single-sugar units that are used for chemically building up the double-unit sugars. *Galactose* occurs only as a constituent of lactose, milk sugar. *Fructose*, or fruit sugar, makes up about 4 to 8 per cent of the weight of fruit and about 40 per cent of honey. It is also known as levulose and is the sweetest of the sugars. The main source of it in our diet is from the breakdown of sucrose, which is now the most important commercial sweetener. However, until sugar cane and sugar beet were refined commercially on a large scale in the nineteenth century, honey was the principal sweetener used in food.

Glucose is the most important of our chemical building blocks. It is found widely in fruit and also occurs in honey (35 per cent w/w), but the main body source is from the breakdown of sucrose and starch, with a little derived from maltose and lactose. It is also known as dextrose or grape sugar. It is not as sweet as sucrose.

The relation between the single- and double-unit sugars and starches is shown in Figure 2.

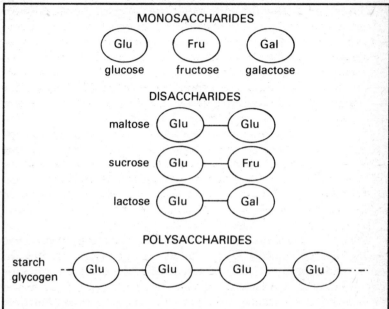

Figure 2 Structures of carbohydrates commonly found in the diet together with glycogen, the body's carbohydrate store

CARBOHYDRATE BIOCHEMISTRY

Digestion of carbohydrates

Carbohydrates are digested in the mouth (where the enzyme *ptyalin* begins its work on the starches) and in the intestine (where, first, *amylase* breaks up starch into two-sugar units; then *maltase*, *sucrase* and *lactase* work on the double units to produce *monosaccharides*).

Food remains in the stomach for three to four hours. Carbohydrates leave there for the intestine before proteins or lipids, which is one reason why we get hungrier more quickly after an all-carbohydrate meal.

Once the starch and sugar have been broken down into glucose units, some of this is used for instant energy and some is stored for use later. In the latter case, the body joins the glucose units back up again to form the polymer *glycogen*, which is then stored mainly in the liver. Glycogen is a branched polymer like starch, and is to animals what starch is to plants – the energy store. We make our glycogen from glucose units; plants make their starch from carbon dioxide and water with the aid of energy from the sun, by a process called *photosynthesis*.

Glucose is probably the most important energy source in the body, providing some 45 per cent of our energy needs. One reason for its importance is that we can extract energy from it even when there is no oxygen present (*anaerobic* conditions). Fatty acids are also an important energy source, especially in the muscles, heart and liver, but their use requires that oxygen is present (*aerobic* conditions).

Glucose can also be converted into fatty acids by some organs, such as the liver, while muscles convert some of the glucose into ATP (*adenosine triphosphate*) to store energy for future use. In times of stress the body can call on glycogen from the liver to provide glucose energy; if the reserves are insufficient, fatty acids can be burnt to provide energy. One of the purposes of aerobic exercise is to burn off fatty acids as an energy source instead of glucose. Stress, in this context, means any increased tension, fear or exercise.

The enzyme *glucagon* is released from the pancreas when blood glucose is low. This stimulates formation of glucose from the glycogen in the liver. Once the glucose level in the blood is high enough, *insulin* from the pancreas shuts off the supply from the liver and also allows the cells to use the circulating glucose more effectively.

In diabetics, who do not manufacture enough insulin of their own, the blood sugar (glucose) is always high but the cells aren't able to use it properly. Insulin increases cellular uptake of glucose and lipids and produces a decrease in free (uncombined) fatty acids in the blood.

The hormones glucagon and insulin do not actually carry out these glucose/glycogen conversions themselves. They simply carry the messages from the pancreas to the liver. They make other enzymes in the liver do the work.

Carbohydrates and diet

When the intake of cane sugar is high, it promotes the manufacture in the body of cholesterol and the fatty acids. There are therefore more lipids in the blood stream. The increased blood sugar level also produces insulin, one of the functions of which is to allow fatty acids greater access to the cells. So with high sugar intake, there is a higher level of fats in the blood and more of them can get into the cells. Fatty cells lead to fatty deposits in the blood vessels; hence the implication of sugar in the development of arteriosclerosis. This is also why you can put on more weight on a high-carbohydrate diet than on a high-fat diet.

Another problem with refined sugar in the diet is that it uses up stores of chromium and vitamin B6 in the body.

ADVERSE REACTIONS

Milk

Many people who suffer from allergies have an adverse reaction to milk or to dairy produce. Leaving aside the possible reaction to the milk proteins for the moment (this will be dealt with in Chapter 18), this could be due to the milk sugar. Milk contains about 5 per cent carbohydrate, most of it in the form of lactose. When this is broken down in the body it forms glucose and galactose. Even for healthy people, too much galactose in the blood is toxic. One of the contributing causes of milk hypersensitivity may be this same galactose intolerance, but at a much lower level. This is not strictly an allergy, as allergies involve interaction between a protein and the body's immune system.

Lactose intolerance is rare amongst Caucasians, but much more common in Asians. Milk and dairy products form no part of the diet of the traditional Chinese, who regard milk as a poison – for many of them, it probably would be. Much of the milk in the USSR is fermented into one of the many forms of yoghurt before it is consumed. In Britain and North America, however, we would find it hard to imagine a diet without milk or cheese.

Occasionally, a baby is born with an inherited genetic defect such that it cannot tolerate galactose at all. The toxicity is so great that milk intake is accompanied in the first instance by vomiting and diarrhoea, and sometimes jaundice as the liver is inflamed. There is a high galactose level in its blood, and it is excreted in the urine; healthy individuals convert galactose into glucose – it never appears in the urine. This problem can be rectified if the condition is detected early enough. Only if the condition is allowed to go untreated does it progress as far as to cause brain damage, which may not be reversible. The condition is known as *galactosemia*.

Fruit

Some people show a surprising intolerance to fruit. There is a little protein even in fruit and vegetables and this may be enough to provoke an allergic response in susceptible individuals. More likely, however, is a reaction against the fructose which the fruit contains, usually to an extent of some 4 to 8 per cent. An excess of fructose can also produce symptoms of toxicity, though it is not as marked as with galactose intolerance. Fructose, too, is normally converted into glucose and burned for energy. If, however, the enzyme *aldolase* in the liver is not sufficiently active, fructose builds up in the blood. This has the same effects as the high sugar levels mentioned previously: high insulin and lipid levels with resulting fatty deposits. In fructose intolerance, sucrose will produce the same clinical effects, as it forms fructose when digested.

INDIGESTIBLE CARBOHYDRATE

In this chapter so far we have taken a look at the digestible carbohydrates – starch and sugar. There is a third carbohydrate in our diet, and a very important one – cellulose.

This is the main chemical ingredient of the fibrous tissue of plants, which ruminant animals can digest and turn into muscle tissue but which we cannot. Cellulose is to plants what protein is to animals – the main structural substance of the organism. In fact, about half the organic carbon in all living matter is in the form of cellulose. The cotton boll is almost 100 per cent pure cellulose. The stems and branches of trees and shrubs are made up of about 50 per cent by weight of cellulose.

Cellulose is made up of a string of glucose units, just like starch and glycogen, but the glucose molecules are joined together in a different way – a way that our bodies cannot unlink. Consequently, for us, cellulose is indigestible. We call it roughage or fibre, and it will be dealt with on its own in Chapter 9 and on pages 52–54.

6
LIPIDS

What are lipids?

Lipids are more varied in their fundamental chemical nature than either the proteins or carbohydrates. They, too, are composed of carbon, hydrogen and oxygen, though they may contain phosphorus or nitrogen as well.

Lipids include fats and oils, and the acids derived from them (the fatty acids); some compounds forming part of the membrane cell wall (which include *phospholipids* like *lecithin*), and chemicals derived from them (like *choline*); and cholesterol. Some people also include the bile acids, which are used to help digest fats, and the fat-soluble vitamins A, D, E and K. The latter are discussed in detail in Chapter 26.

With their diverse chemical structure, lipids play a variety of roles in body chemistry. Unlike starches and proteins, the lipids are not polymers. They do not dissolve in water but are soluble in certain organic solvents like chloroform or carbon tetrachloride (one of the liquids used in dry cleaning or domestic stain removers).

Lipids in food

The main dietary sources of lipids are milk and other dairy products like butter and cheese; nuts; meat; oily fish like tuna, eels and mackerel; eggs; and the fats and oils used in cooking.

Digestion of lipids

Lipids are digested in the intestine (by a group of enzymes known as *lipases*). In order to be digested they have first to be dissolved, or at least dispersed into small droplets. Digestive juice in the stomach is highly acidic and water-based, and the lipids are insoluble. Once the food enters the small intestine it starts encountering digestive juices which are neutral or even alkaline. These help the fat to dissolve. (That's why cleaning fluids in the home are made alkaline with caustic soda or ammonia – to dissolve grease.)

The problem of having a water-based gastric juice still has to be overcome, since the lipids would not be really soluble even if the solution were alkaline. To achieve this, the liver manufactures steroidal *bile acids*

29

out of cholesterol. These are shipped off to the gall bladder for storage. When lipids enter the intestine, the gall bladder contracts and sodium or potassium salts of the bile acids are injected into the intestine to be mixed with the food. These bile salts act like detergents in washing-up liquid: they enable lipids to dissolve, or at least to disperse, forming small droplets. The total surface area of these tiny droplets is so very much greater than that of the large drops that the digestive enzymes have more opportunity to go to work.

Once the lipids have been digested they are processed along a different route from that used for proteins and carbohydrates. Products from the latter are passed through the intestinal wall into the blood stream. The constituents of lipids are channelled through the centre of little projections (*villi*) on the wall of the intestine direct into the lymphatic system, the body's reserve fluid supply which complements the blood stream.

FATS AND OILS

The difference between a *fat* and an *oil* is that fats are solids and oils are liquids at room temperature. This difference in physical appearance arises because of a difference in chemical composition, as we shall see shortly.

In order that fats can be transported around the blood stream they are joined together (*conjugated*) with proteins. Most of the lipids in the blood stream occur in the form of these water-soluble lipoproteins.

The circulating lipid is then deposited in the *fat depots* of the body, which are located under the skin, in the palms of the hands and soles of the feet, behind the eyes and around the kidneys. Women have additional fat depots in the breasts and on the inside of the legs at the top of the thighs. The ready use of the fat from around the eyes when we are ill gives us the characteristic gaunt appearance of the invalid. The tissue where fat is stored is called *adipose tissue*.

As well as insulating us against the cold, the fat layer under the skin cushions our bones and internal organs to protect them against injury: so there are at least two benefits of a fat covering!

A third use of fat is as an energy source. When they are burned, fatty acids produce twice the number of calories that can be obtained from the same weight of glucose. They are a vital part of the body's fuel supply.

A fat is made up of an acid joined together with *glycerol* (or glycerine), which is a member of the family of alcohols. It, too, can be converted quite easily in three steps into glucose and hence used in this way as an energy source. The reverse change of glucose into glycerol is equally easy for the body to carry out and provides one route for the conversion of carbohydrates into lipids. This is one of the reasons why people put on weight as fat by eating carbohydrates.

Oils are also derived from glycerol; the difference between these and fats is in the nature of the acid, and this is what we must now look at in more detail.

FATTY ACIDS

The acids which are found in fats, joined chemically to glycerol, are called, as one would expect, *fatty acids*. The simplest member of the series, formic acid, gets its name from the Latin word *formica*, which means 'ant'. It is the acid injected into us by ant bites and nettle stings, and is found in the body only as derivatives – parts of other larger molecules.

The next simplest member of the series is acetic acid, which is found in vinegar. This exists in the body in its charged form, the acetate ion. It is the starting point for many of the body's chemical reactions, including the formation of cholesterol.

Animal fats yield more complicated fatty acids, such as *butyric acid* (from milk fat and butter) and *stearic acid* (from beef, pork, mutton or lamb suet). Fatty acids of this type are also found occasionally in vegetable oils: for example, palm oil yields *palmitic acid*. Acids such as these are described as *saturated*, which means that the carbon atoms in the acids have no reserve combining power to take up hydrogen atoms chemically. Although they are sometimes found in plants, saturated fatty acids are characteristic of animal produce.

Vegetable oils tend to contain mainly *unsaturated acids*, that is, compounds in which the carbon atoms do still have some reserve combining power to take hydrogens on board. You may well see the names of some of these as ingredients in cooking oils or margarines; examples are *oleic acid* (olive oil), *erucic acid* (rapeseed and cod-liver oil) and *nervonic acid* (brain-tissue and fish-liver oils).

Some of the acids which are obtained from oils have still greater reserve combining power than the ones listed above, such as *linoleic acid* (in linseed and corn oil), *linolenic acid* (in soya and poppy-seed oil) and *arachidonic acid* (in peanuts). These are called *polyunsaturated acids*.

Do not worry about all these complicated chemical names. They are given here just for reference so that you will recognize them if you should come across them on supermarket shelves when all ingredients have to be listed in foodstuffs, by law.

The term 'fatty acids' is used by nutritionists to describe any acid derived from a fat or oil. The term is used a little more restrictedly by chemists to denote only the saturated acids.

Because the unsaturated acids tend to have lower melting points than the naturally occurring saturated acids, the vegetable lipids are usually liquids (oils), while those from animal sources are more often solids (fats) at room temperature. Unsaturated acids are unstable even in the body, and one role of vitamin E is to prolong their life and function.

Linoleic, linolenic and arachidonic acids used to be known collectively as vitamin F, though this term is rarely used nowadays. They are called *essential fatty acids*, a term that is still widely used, because they are necessary for health, but they must be taken directly in the diet since they cannot be made by the body. This is the same use of the word 'essential' as we met with amino acids in Chapter 4.

Unsaturation in fatty acids is important in allowing them to function as oxidizing agents. This means that the carbon atoms can use their reserve combining power to attach on to more hydrogen atoms. This is a vital property in their biological action. Saturated acids are not able to do this since all of the carbon atoms are joined up to as many hydrogens as they can cope with. The reason that polyunsaturated fats are so important is that they can take care of even more hydrogen atoms than unsaturated acids. Because of this property, polyunsaturates are also less stable and need to be 'protected' by compounds such as vitamin E.

Another use of unsaturated fatty acids in the body is the provision of components for the lipid complexes, like *lecithin*, found in the membrane cell wall.

In addition to lining and eventually blocking our blood vessels, saturated fats interfere with the way the body utilizes unsaturated fatty acids.

We shall now look at another major biological transformation involving these compounds.

Prostaglandins

One of the functions of unsaturated fatty acids, once they have been extracted from the lipids in our diet, is to act as starting material for the formation of *prostaglandins*. The first of these was isolated in the 1930s from, as the name suggests, the male prostate gland. Research work on the prostaglandins has increased in the past two decades and they are now known to be components of many different types of tissue.

Amongst the functions of prostaglandins in the body are the regulation of menstruation and conception, inducing childbirth, lowering blood pressure, inhibiting blood clotting, and promoting inflammation. As aspirin inhibits inflammation, part of its action in the treatment of arthritis may be its interaction with prostaglandin, in addition to its pain-killing effect.

Prostaglandins seem to act in modifying the effects of hormones (see

Chapter 10), in much the same way as some vitamins, acting as cofactors, modify the action of enzymes. So conversion to prostaglandins is a significant role for the unsaturated fatty acids in our diet.

CHOLESTEROL

Much has been said in recent years about the role of cholesterol in diseases of the heart and blood vessels (*arteriosclerosis*). This has tended to produce the view that cholesterol is in some way toxic to the body, which is not at all the case.

The body continually manufactures cholesterol in the liver, starting from acetate. The normal blood level of cholesterol is 150 to 250 mg per 100 ml of blood. As there are about 6 l (10½ pints) of blood in the body, this means there are about 12 g of cholesterol just circulating in the blood. Cholesterol is also a component of cell membranes and there are several grams more located there.

The level of cholesterol in the blood does not seem to vary significantly with the amount we get in our diet. So if we eat more cholesterol, either the rate at which it is made in the liver slows down, or the rate at which it is converted into other things speeds up. A third possibility is that it may be deposited as fatty lining (*plaque*) in the blood vessels.

A certain amount of cholesterol in the body is therefore essential. It forms the starting point for the formation of bile acids, which help fats form a suspension in the digestive juices so that they can be broken down more easily by enzymes (*lipases*).

By another series of reactions, cholesterol is converted into the sex hormones which are necessary for normal sexual activity.

Still more cholesterol is needed to form the hormones of the outer part of the adrenal gland. This region is known as the adrenal cortex and its secretions are called *adrenocortical hormones*. One of the best known is *cortisol*, used in the treatment of arthritis. Some of the male sex hormones are produced here (others in the sex glands), and so is the steroid hormone *aldosterone*, which is involved in the salt and water balance in the body.

From this it will be clear that, far from being toxic, cholesterol is an integral part of the healthy body. It seems, however, that we can manufacture all we need and there is no necessity for us to include cholesterol at all in our diet. If we do so to excess it seems to predispose us to arterial disease, but the relationship is by no means clear as yet.

The main food sources of cholesterol are eggs (which contain about 450 mg per 100 g/3½ oz, or 225 mg per large egg) and butter (230 mg per 100 g/3½ oz, or 2.5 mg per generously buttered slice of bread).

LIPIDS AND DIET

Since fat can be formed from other lipids, from proteins or (most easily) from carbohydrates, either a high-fat diet or a high carbohydrate intake will increase the incorporation of fat into the tissues and produce weight gain.

We have already discussed the interconversion of glycerol (from fat) and glucose. Unfortunately, there are other mechanisms at work which contribute to weight gain on a high-sugar diet. Although it may be a curse to slimmers, it is a clinically interesting paradox that you can gain more weight on a high-sugar diet than on a high-fat diet. Let's look at some of the other reasons why.

For one thing, granulated sugar (sucrose) increases the lipid-forming enzyme activity much more than glucose or starch. Thus, more sugar means more circulating lipids.

Furthermore, the high blood sugar levels mean high insulin levels, an increase in blood glucose, and still more glucose converted into fat. In addition, the elevated levels of insulin promote entry and absorption of fat into the cells.

On the other hand, a high-fat diet, if sugar intake is low, produces low insulin and low blood glucose levels, and less fat absorbed into the cells. More fat will then be used up to satisfy energy requirements.

By this argument, a large meal with increased insulin and glucose in the blood will produce more weight gain than the same food taken in smaller meals, which keeps the glucose and insulin levels lower. The weight gain from a large meal will be greater if the fat content of the meal is high. So the message for slimmers is this: if you eat fatty foods, eat them on their own, a little at a time, and without sugar. Those cream cakes eaten at the end of a large meal, or with two or three cups of sugar-rich drink, do far more damage than the same cream cake on its own in the middle of the morning or afternoon with a cup of sugarless tea or coffee.

Whenever alcohol is taken, lipid deposition in the liver is increased. This becomes more of a problem with regular drinkers. Two or three glasses of wine or their alcoholic equivalent each day may do wonders for dissolving cholesterol out of the arteries, but the problem is that they do much more damage by depositing most of it back in the liver. Terminal inflammation of the liver (*cirrhosis*) is almost always accompanied by a 'fatty liver'.

7
VITAMINS:
an introduction

The discovery of vitamins

In addition to the macronutrients discussed in the last four chapters – water, protein, carbohydrates and lipids – there are two vital sets of micronutrients that are required for health: vitamins and minerals. We shall take a brief look at these in this and the next chapter, and consider each in detail in Chapters 26 and 27.

When vitamins were first discovered – and that was only at the turn of the century – they were named by being assigned letters of the alphabet. They were detected as substances which, if they were absent from the diet, would produce symptoms of disease: they were anti-disease factors.

The first to emerge was a substance which prevented a nervous disease called beriberi, and it was thought to belong to the class of chemical compounds called amines – an essential or vital amine.

It was Casimir Funk, a Polish biochemist working in the Lister Institute in London, who, in 1911, first coined the name 'vitamine'. At that time only four of these disease-preventing micronutrients were recognized: those curing the symptoms of beriberi, pellagra, rickets and scurvy. The one which prevented beriberi was called 'vitamine B'.

Since then 'vitamine B' has been shown to be a mixture of many different chemical compounds, each of which has a distinctive role in the body. Several of these components are not even amines, in fact, so the word is now usually spelt 'vitamin' without the final 'e'.

What are vitamins?

There are seven vitamin groups which have so far been distinguished: A, B, C, D, E, F and K. Of these, only vitamin C is a single chemical compound; the rest are mixtures of two or more substances. For this reason they are often referred to now by common chemical names so that it is quite clear which compound is being talked about (for vitamin C, of course, it doesn't matter). The different members of each vitamin group tend to be derived from similar sources and are used to prevent similar diseases, though there is more variation with the vitamin B group than with others. For this reason, we generally use the letters when we refer to

35

the sources or diseases, and the chemical names when we want to talk about quantities of specific compounds as nutrients or their role in the body.

Vitamins B and C are soluble in water, but the others are fat-soluble vitamins. Water-soluble vitamins are generally absorbed direct into the blood stream and any quantities that are not used are excreted by the kidneys into the urine. Comparatively few are stored in the body. Water-soluble vitamins are used as *coenzymes*, assisting in control of the body's chemistry (see Chapter 10). Fat-soluble vitamins (A, D, E, F and K) pass into the blood or lymph system, and excesses are either stored or excreted through the liver into the faeces.

It is essential that we get adequate amounts of vitamins B and C daily, and it is unlikely that high doses will be toxic. In the case of fat-soluble vitamins, however, the body maintains some reserve of most of these, and daily intake significantly higher than the RDA values should not be encouraged as the result may prove toxic.

The vitamin content of food

In the chapters on macronutrients it was possible to give some idea of how much protein, say, or fibre we can get from particular foods. With vitamins and minerals, the amount in any one food varies greatly, particularly with the least stable vitamins: A, C and E. One orange, for example, may contain less than 10 mg or as much as 100 mg of vitamin C. To get a generous daily dose of the vitamin, do we eat one or ten oranges? Vitamins are also frequently destroyed by storage, cooking or other methods of processing food. For this reason, quantities of micronutrients in food are rarely given in Chapters 26 and 27, where vitamins and minerals are discussed in more detail, since they have little meaning. Instead, I have simply listed the food sources in which the micronutrient is most abundant. To get the best of the vitamin (and mineral) content of fruit and vegetables, they should always be eaten fresh and raw, if possible.

8

MINERALS:
an introduction

What are minerals?

When scientists use the word 'mineral' they usually mean those crystalline chemical units that make up the rocks of the earth. Nutritionists use the word in a different sense. To them a mineral is an inorganic element essential to good health. Carbon, hydrogen, oxygen and nitrogen are excluded because they form the main bulk of our tissues.

Unlike organic substances, which get burned for energy or transformed into completely different types of compound, the inorganic salts remain in the body as ions (charged atoms or groups of atoms), often in exactly the same form through several biochemical processes. They are not degraded; they remain in our bodies until they are excreted.

The mineral content of food

Although the mineral content of food cannot be destroyed, it may be removed during processing (including cooking) from the portion of the food that we eat. The refining of sugar and grain, for example, takes away most of the valuable minerals which are found in raw sugar and whole-grain cereals. Unenriched white flour and white sugar contain no nutrients, just energy. In cooking, some of the mineral content of vegetables passes into the water in which they are prepared. The mineral content of food also depends to a great extent on the nature of the soil in which plants were grown or on which animals were grazed.

Minerals in the body

Once inside our bodies, some minerals move around most of the time as individual atoms or ions (like the sodium ion). Other elements (like phosphorus) are always combined with one or more different atoms (in the case of phosphorus this is oxygen, which forms a phosphate ion). There are still others that may exist either as ions or as part of bigger organic molecules, like sulphur in the amino acid cysteine, phosphorus in ATP, cobalt in vitamin B12, or iron in haemoglobin.

Some of these elements are needed in relatively large quantities of several grams daily (macrominerals); some are needed in only tiny amounts of a few milli- or micrograms (microminerals).

A further division of these inorganic mineral elements can be made into metals and non-metals. The complete list of these considered in detail in Chapter 27 is shown in Table 3.

Table 3   Mineral elements known to be essential for health

	Metals	Non-metals
Macrominerals	sodium	phosphorus
	potassium	sulphur
	magnesium	chlorine
	calcium	
Microminerals	iron	selenium
	zinc	fluorine
	copper	iodine
	cobalt	
	chromium	
	manganese	
	molybdenum	

Notes
1   The metals form positively charged ions (*cations*).
2   The non-metals form negatively charged ions (*anions*).
3   Some elements may form individual ions or they may be part of a bigger organic molecule.

9
FIBRE

Roughage, or dietary fibre, is the last of the food components we need to consider. It is not a nutrient in the usual sense, as we do not take body-building material out of it. However, it is certainly essential for health in assisting the elimination of the waste products of the body's chemical reactions.

Fibre is the structural tissue of plants. It is made up largely of the carbohydrate *cellulose*, with other carbohydrates like *hemicellulose* and *pectin* (which is used to make jam set), and the non-carbohydrate *lignin*. Cud-chewing animals (ruminants) can digest cellulose but we can't. It is acted on by bacteria in the lower part of the gut (large intestine), where it is mixed with the waste products of our food. Excess moisture is removed at this stage and the whole mass compacted before excretion.

Cellulose is to plants what protein is to animals: it is the very stuff of the structure of the living organism. Most of the carbohydrate in plants is starch; the cellulose component of vegetables, fruit and cereal grains is only a small but vital proportion: usually less than 5 per cent and often less than 1 per cent.

The grains of cereals consist of three parts. The main central bulk is the *endosperm*, composed of starch and protein. The outer *bran* layer is largely cellulose. The *germ*, made up of both types of carbohydrate, starch and cellulose, with a little protein, is rich in unsaturated fats and thiamin (vitamin B1). Wheat bran contains up to 10 per cent cellulose and is the richest source of dietary fibre.

White rice and white flour have little dietary value except to provide calories. If the rice is eaten as a pudding, the milk contributes protein, fat, vitamins and minerals. White bread is generally enhanced with calcium (as the carbonate) vitamins, and now some bakeries add additional fibre, but these are the only nutrients.

Brown bread is no better nutritionally than white unless it has whole grain added to it. For example, a slice of wholemeal bread provides 2.5 to 3 g of fibre, but ordinary brown or white bread contains only about one-tenth of this amount.

One of the best sources of dietary fibre nowadays is breakfast cereal. These are usually enriched with one or more of their natural

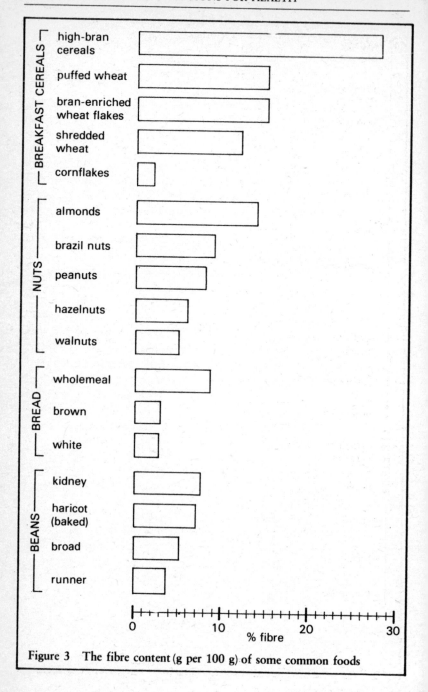

Figure 3   The fibre content (g per 100 g) of some common foods

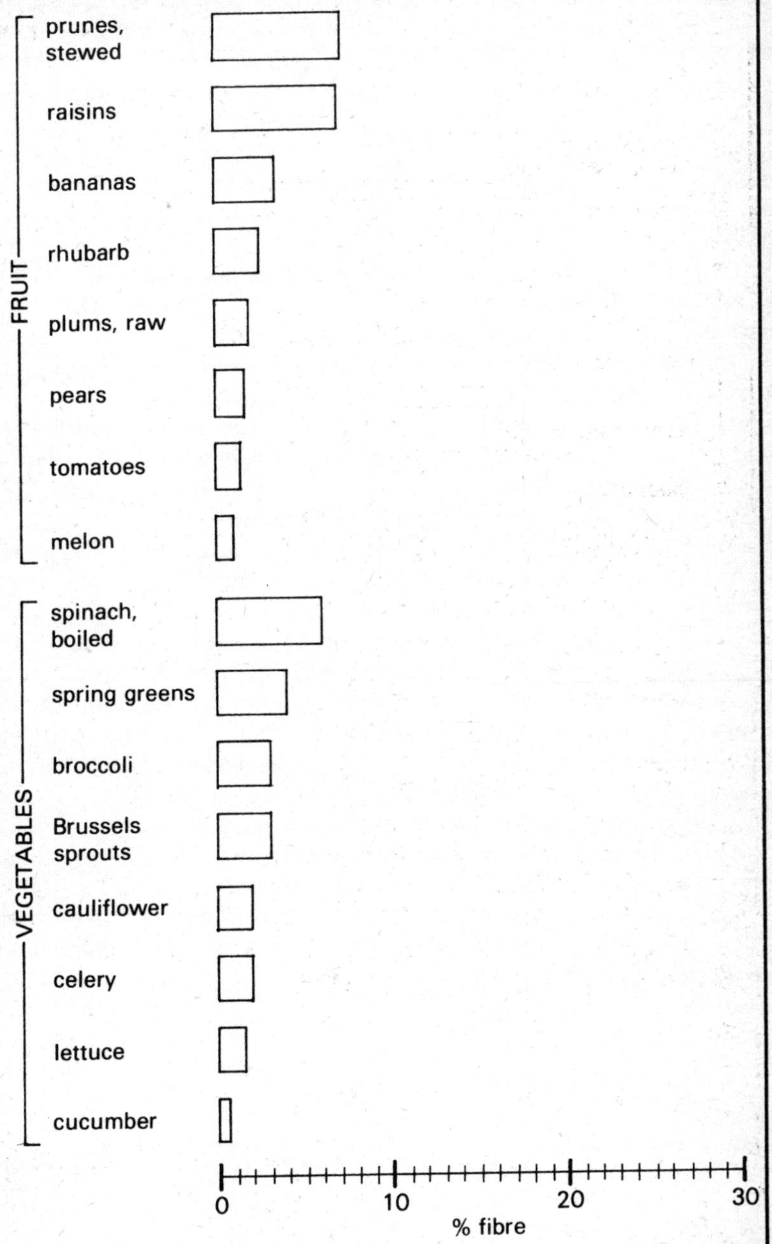

Figure 3 *continued*

components, which may have been partially lost in the processing, and minerals, vitamins and bran are also added to many. High-bran cereal contains about 20 to 30 per cent fibre; puffed wheat or whole-wheat flakes, especially if the latter are enriched with bran, contain 12 to 16 per cent fibre; porridge contains about 7 per cent fibre; and most other breakfast cereals contain 5 per cent fibre or less. If you are partial to corn flakes or puffed rice cereal, try mixing them with some of the high-bran products: this will give a completely different taste and will boost the fibre quota.

A generously heaped cereal bowl of bran-enriched wheat flakes weighs about 60 g (2 oz) and will provide 9 g of fibre (obviously the precise weights depend upon the size of your bowl!). The same bulk of volume of puffed wheat, which is just as rich in fibre content, weight-for-weight, weighs only 30 g (1 oz) and therefore gives you rather less than 5 g of fibre. But this same bulk quantity of high-bran cereal, which many people might find somewhat indigestible, weighs about 120 g (4¼ oz) and therefore provides nearly 35 g of fibre – most of your day's requirement.

The fibre content of fruit and vegetables is usually less than 5 per cent of their weight, and often less than 1 per cent. Obviously you have to eat much more of these if you do not get sufficient fibre from whole-grain cereals. Most common salad ingredients (tomatoes, lettuce, cucumber and cress) have little fibre, but the much-maligned baked (haricot) bean is quite a good source of fibre (about 7 per cent), although the canned variety in sauce does contain a significant amount of added sugar (about 4 per cent). Other pulses (split lentils, kidney beans, broad beans and runner beans) have 3 to 7 per cent fibre. Nuts are much better: most contain 7 to 14 per cent dietary fibre.

Thus, most cereals and nuts are a good source of fibre and should make up a significant portion of the diet each day; fruit and vegetables do provide you with some fibre, but not enough to make up the daily fibre quota on their own (see Figure 3). You will find more about roughage on pages 52–54.

ENZYMES AND HORMONES

ENZYMES

Biochemical reactions in the body are controlled by *enzymes* – proteins made from amino acids which, in turn, are produced by digestion of the protein food we eat. All enzymes are proteins but not all proteins are enzymes.

We need enzymes to make our chemical reactions happen at a lower temperature. If the enzymes were not there, the chemicals in our bodies would never react appreciably at body temperature. Enzymes speed up or slow down chemical reactions: they act as a control mechanism (what the chemists call *catalysts*). They work by increasing or decreasing the energy (*activation energy*) which chemicals need in order to rearrange themselves before they change over to take on their new chemical partners. Enzymes themselves are not used up but are recycled for continual use.

The body has mechanisms for turning on and off the manufacture of enzymes, depending on our requirements. This was discovered as long ago as 1900 and was extensively investigated by the French biologist Jacques Monod, one of the great names in biochemistry, who was awarded the Nobel Prize for Medicine in 1965 as a result of his work.

We have seen already that lipids are not polymers but relatively small molecules; starches, although they are polymers, are made up of only one type of chemical building block, which can be joined up in various ways. This means that only a limited number of different types of molecular arrangement can be made out of lipids or carbohydrates.

For this reason, proteins have been chosen for the job as enzymes in our bodies. If we start with twenty different amino acids, we can make literally millions of proteins by joining these up in various ways. This gives us enormous possibilities for making individual protein enzymes for every job. Each protein has its own unique three-dimensional shape which is determined by the nature and order of the amino acids. This enables those proteins which act as enzymes to be very selective about the compounds they react with. There is usually a region of the enzyme specifically shaped for the reacting molecules: this is known as the lock-

and-key mechanism, and it gives enzymes their high *specificity* – one reaction, one enzyme. We therefore need many thousands of enzymes to control our overall metabolism.

If we lack the ability to make a particular enzyme, there is little we can do about it from a dietary point of view. However, the absence of certain essential minerals or vitamins in the diet may prevent the body from making an enzyme even though the system for its manufacture works perfectly well. In these circumstances, addition of the mineral or vitamin to the diet usually gets things working normally again.

There are very many enzymes which either contain a metallic mineral atom as part of their structure or require the presence of a mineral or vitamin in order to be able to do their work. A non-protein substance, the presence of which is required for an enzyme to function, is called a *cofactor*. If the cofactor is a metal ion, it is called an *activator*; if it is another organic molecule, like those derived from the water-soluble vitamins, the cofactor is called a *coenzyme*.

Sometimes a complete enzyme can be injected or taken orally, like pepsin swallowed with food to aid digestion, but usually the absence of an enzyme means we have to avoid certain types of food. We cannot treat disorders like phenylketonuria or galactosemia, for example, by injecting the appropriate enzymes from animals or other humans, because the body would develop antibodies to them and make them inactive by rejection.

HORMONES

Fortunately, this situation does not apply for many of the hormones, which are usually much smaller molecules. Whereas enzymes control individual reactions, hormones influence whole systems or processes which occur at a site in the body remote from where the hormones are made.

Hormones may be proteins, parts of proteins (*polypeptides*) or steroids. They are made in the body by a special set of glands (the *endocrine glands*) and are secreted directly into the blood stream so that they can be despatched to their target organ. All the glands are under the direct control of a master gland (the *pituitary gland*) at the base of the brain.

Thyroid hormones

Occasionally, we can influence our hormone levels directly through diet. If, for example, we have insufficient iodine in our food, the appropriate gland in the neck, the thyroid gland, cannot make enough of its hormone (*thyroxine*). As a result, a person develops protruding eyes and a swollen neck (the symptoms of goitre). In this case the condition is usually reversed quite easily by administration of iodine in the diet, assuming it was a lack of this mineral that caused the problem. If it was due to some other hormone imbalance, however, dietary regulation is ineffective, as is the case with most hormone deficiencies.

The thyroid controls the overall rate of biochemical reactions in the body. When the thyroid is overactive (*hyperthyroidism*), a person will be slim, and agitated and restless in manner. When it is too sluggish (*hypothyroidism*), a person will gain weight, perhaps to the point of obesity, and will be lethargic. Only rarely, however, is this the cause of overweight; more often obesity is due to overeating or lack of exercise.

Sex hormones

It has long been held that certain foods (aphrodisiacs) are capable of stimulating our sex drive or *libido* by their action on the sex hormones. These hormones control the onset of puberty, the menopause, the menstrual cycle, the various physiological changes associated with childbirth and suckling, and all the sexual changes which occur through our lives. Although vitamin E is necessary for the health of the sex cells in some animals, there is no reliable evidence, however, that it has any beneficial effects on sex drive in humans.

It is also these sex hormones which are directly affected by the administration of oral contraceptives, although this is the action of drugs not foods. One component of the contraceptives, progesterone, increases the thickness of the plug of mucus (the *cervical plug*) at the entrance of the womb; normally it prepares the walls of the uterus to receive the ovum if it has been fertilized on its journey down the Fallopian tube. Other contraceptive hormones, oestrogens, allow most of the physiological changes associated with menstruation to proceed, but prevent the release of the egg cell (*ovulation*) from the female sex glands (*ovaries*) each month.

Low blood progesterone levels in the second half of the menstrual cycle also account for the symptoms known as pre-menstrual tension (PMT) or the pre-menstrual syndrome (PMS) in nearly half of those women who have this problem. Treatment with 40 to 80 mg of pyridoxine (vitamin B6) daily has been found to help many PMT sufferers, though the mechanism of action is not clear.

Apart from this one instance, however, there are no established examples of any components of diet directly affecting sex hormone levels and therefore sex drive. If lettuce leaves or oysters do have any aphrodisiac effect, the biochemical mechanism is not known.

Pancreatic hormones

The *insulin* and *glucagon* secreted by the pancreas to control the amount of glucose in the blood are also hormones. In many cases, as we have seen, we cannot utilize an enzyme or organ from another animal, even if it does the same job in the human body, because of rejection. With the hormone insulin, however, we are fortunate that the molecule is relatively small, and the differences between human and pig or cow insulin are so slight that we can use these animals as sources of the hormone for diabetics.

These hormones are affected by diet only in so far as they do what they are supposed to do in our bodies by responding to the level of sugar intake. It appears that eating excessive amounts of sugar wears out this delicate control mechanism, leading to obesity and diabetes. It has not been established with certainty whether it is the high blood sugar or the artificial insulin in diabetics which gives rise to the secondary symptoms of opacity of the eye lens (*cataract*), retinal damage, and gangrene of the feet.

Adrenal hormones

Other hormones (*adrenaline* and *noradrenaline*), secreted by the central portion of glands located just above the kidneys (the *adrenal medulla*), control our reactions to stress: loss of colour or blushing, sweating, palpitations, increased breathing rate and raised blood pressure. Certain foods, like tea or coffee, will stimulate their release.

The outer portion of these same glands (the *adrenal cortex*) makes steroid hormones which affect the balance of salts (*electrolytes*) in our blood stream. There are two main hormones (*cortisol* and *aldosterone*): one of these (*cortisol*) and a close chemical relative (*cortisone*) are used to treat arthritis, which is now thought to be due to a disorder in the biochemistry of these salts. This results in inflammation or deposition of calcium in the joints. Sodium and potassium in our diet will affect the secretion of these hormones.

Thus, although the secretion or release of some hormones is greatly affected by specific foods, we cannot generally influence their manufacture in the body by alterations of diet if the biological equipment for making them is out of order. In these cases, however, we can often inject comparable hormones from animals other than man.

11
DIET

Introduction

Sometimes the word 'diet' is used to mean more or less the same as food, but the context is such that it usually implies some restriction in our selection. There are now many types of diet available, all designed for better health, and many for weight loss, and in this chapter we'll take a look at ten of them. There are several that I, personally, would not recommend, but you must make up your own mind from the details given. These will tell you something of the restrictions involved in each diet and the problems you may encounter. My own recommendations for weight loss or gain and health maintenance are given in Chapter 14, 'The Good-health Plan'.

THE VEGETARIAN DIET

There are many variations in vegetarian diet but its followers typically eat fish, eggs, milk and other dairy produce, but no meat. Some vegetarians omit only red meat but do eat poultry; some exclude one or more of these other foods.

People adopt vegetarian diets either for health, moral or religious reasons. For example, the Seventh Day Adventists, a North American religious group founded in 1860, are strict vegetarians. As these and other devotees of vegetarianism have shown, a diet without meat has no ill effects on the body as long as there is a balanced intake of essential nutrients from other food sources.

Meat is a concentrated protein source (10 to 20 per cent of the total weight is protein), but so are many other foods, particularly fish and nuts, eggs, legumes and avocado. The lipid content of meat is mainly saturated fat and the body is better off without it. Tongue, pork and lamb generally have a higher fat content than beef.

Meat is usually hung for ten to thirty days after killing and before retailing; it may be hung even longer at the butcher's shop. The purpose of this is to allow tenderizing of the meat by the action of protein-breaking (*proteolytic*) enzymes, which work on the muscle tissue to make the meat more digestible for humans. The process is sometimes assisted by the injection of *papain* into the live animal before slaughter so that this protein-breaking enzyme reaches all its tissues. The enzyme is active only in the temperature range of 55 to 71°C (131 to 160°F), achieved as the meat is cooked.

Sex hormones and antibiotics are injected into animals or added to their feed in order to accelerate growth and produce a higher proportion of lean tissue. The theory is that these chemicals are all broken down by the animal's metabolic processes before slaughter.

In order to prevent the growth of a highly toxic bacterium (*Clostridium botulinum*), which produces a frequently fatal disease called *botulism*, meat is preserved by the addition of a small quantity of sodium nitrite or nitrate, or potassium nitrite. Almost all packaged and tinned meats have these additives (E249, 250 and 251). Unfortunately, in destroying the bacteria, nitrites may be partially converted into nitrosamines, known cancer-forming chemicals (*carcinogens*). The same change may occur in the gut during digestion. The hazard of cancer formation has to be balanced against the risk of botulism if the chemical were not used. A meat-free diet avoids both!

The blood in meat is a good source of iron – but so are some beans, nuts, fruits and lentils. Brewer's yeast contains about twice as much iron, weight-for-weight, as most meat sources; the problem here is that it is not really practicable to eat the same quantity of yeast as you would meat.

Vitamin B12 is found most abundantly in meat, especially offal, but there are alternative dietary sources as it also occurs to a lesser extent in eggs and milk, as well as in brewer's yeast.

Finally, meat is a rich source of bacteria and infection, in the form of germs which are not always killed off by the cooking, especially if the meat is eaten rare. It may also contain a selection of other chemicals which we can well do without. This in itself is not really sufficient reason for avoiding a meat diet, however, since many other foods nowadays are packaged with additives, and many may be contaminated by environmental pollutants: we have no way of knowing for certain.

Provided they have a balanced diet and ensure they obtain a variety of protein, and adequate iron and B12, vegetarians may well be better off nutritionally than those who place no restrictions on their diet.

THE VEGAN DIET

Vegans eat no meat, fish, eggs, milk or dairy produce, or any food of animal origin. Again, this more extreme form of vegetarianism may be practised either for health or religious reasons. As a result of the dietary restrictions, vegans are in a more difficult position nutritionally than other vegetarians.

It is difficult for vegans to get enough calcium without dairy foods. Hard water or mineral waters may be good alternative sources, but in soft-water districts, the best food sources are brewer's yeast, watercress and soya. In Britain and the US white bread (but not wholemeal bread) now contains about 0.1 per cent (w/w) calcium in the form of calcium carbonate.

Calcium absorption in the body requires vitamin D, and the main sources of this are all foods which the vegan does not eat: oily fish like mackerel, eels, herrings and kippers; butter and margarine; and eggs. Without a vitamin supplement, vegans have difficulty in getting enough vitamin D, however varied their diet. In sunny climates, the action of sunlight on the skin may produce enough vitamin D for health, but this would rarely be the case in Britain, northern continental Europe, or Canada.

The same foods that provide vitamin D also have vitamin A in them. Fortunately, there are other vegetarian foods containing a compound known as *carotene*, which the body can convert easily into vitamin A. Whereas the daily requirement of vitamin A is 1 mg, that of beta-carotene is 6 mg and that of other carotenoids is 12 mg because only a portion of these compounds is absorbed and converted into vitamin A in the body. Carotene and other carotenoids are found in carrots, tomatoes, apricots, sweet potatoes and most red- or yellow-coloured fruit and vegetables (except oranges, which owe their yellow colour to xanthophyll).

Vitamin E, which also occurs in eggs and animal fats, is found abundantly in wheatgerm and vegetable oils, so this creates no problem for those on a vegan diet. But vegans do have a problem in obtaining enough vitamin B12 in their diet, since the principal sources are meat, offal and, to a lesser extent, eggs and milk. The most acceptable dietary alternative is brewer's yeast, but a tablet supplement is recommended for vegans.

The comments made about the potential lack of iron in a meat-free vegetarian diet also apply to vegans (see page 48).

Because so many foods are excluded on a vegan diet, and others are taken in greater quantities than normal, there is an increased tendency for allergic or hypersensitivity reactions to develop towards such foods as wheat, carrots and oranges. If additional foods have to be excluded from the diet on allergy grounds, adequate nutrition becomes a very real problem for vegans.

THE FASTING DIET

This is promoted as the ultimate diet plan. Quite simply, it demands no eating at all. With no food, you have no calorie input, and very soon you start burning off body fat to keep you going. At least, that's the theory. As usual, there are advantages and disadvantages of the method.

If you are reasonably healthy, apart from being overweight, fasting *for a short period* (two or three days) will do you no harm and is the quickest way to lose a little weight.

Fasting as a religious atonement is thousands of years old. It is an integral part of the twenty-four-hour-long Jewish observance of Yom Kippur, the holiest of holy days. The Muslim faith, Islam, founded in the seventh century, has a month-long fast to accompany the Ramadan. Only the young, the old, the sick, and expectant or nursing mothers are allowed dispensation from the fast. Liquid nourishments, including soups, are allowed for everyone, however.

There is ample evidence, then, that *for people in good health* even extended fasting is not harmful. It gives the body a chance to rest and recharge itself. It is certainly the most effective method of losing a great deal of weight quickly. It is possible to lose up to 2.25 kg (5 lb) a day for the first two or three days of a fast, though most people will not lose as much as this. The weight you shed will depend on a number of factors which we will go into as we look at some of the disadvantages of this kind of diet.

First, it requires just as much willpower not to eat food at all as it does to avoid all those tempting goodies when you're on any other diet. Once a fast is established (usually about three or four days), the stomach contracts and the secretion of digestive enzymes is reduced. It's those first three or four days that are the problem.

When you fast, you burn up all your reserves of glucose, so the body looks around for something else to burn for energy. It has two choices – fat or protein. If you are going to persuade it to burn fat you have to take a significant amount of exercise every day during the fast, otherwise your body will start converting protein, that is, muscle tissue, into glucose. Most people find it difficult enough to maintain a nine-to-five routine on a fast, at home or at work, let alone find the energy for exercise. The exercise needs to be regular, through the day; it must be extensive, that is, using as many of the different muscles of the body as possible; and it must make your heart and lungs work harder – *aerobic exercise* – in order to burn off fat.

When the fast is over, you have to start eating again, if you don't want to expire completely. If, when you go back on food, you resume bad eating habits, you will regain all the weight you lost, probably more, and the wrong sort. In order to lose weight and stay healthy you have to adopt good eating habits whether you fast or not.

When you are fasting for more than a couple of days, the body's metabolism slows down. When you start eating again, unless you introduce food gradually, your digestion cannot cope and some of the excess goes on as flab instead of being converted into fuel or muscle. This might replace the good solid muscle tissue you had before fasting and which was burned up for energy.

When you come off a fast of more than two days, it is *essential*, therefore, that you start slowly and take as long to build up to full food intake as you were fasting. You must start with small meals, high in carbohydrate, low in protein. During a fast, your body gears itself to burn amino acids for energy, instead of converting them into protein. When they are burned, amino acids form ammonia, and these amino-acid-burning enzymes will go to work if you eat a lot of protein. At the very least this will give you indigestion. In an extreme case you can even die from ammonia poisoning, as happened to some prisoners-of-war released after the Second World War, who were fed nourishing, high-protein diets.

It is important in fasting to be sure that you keep up the input of salts (*electrolytes*) into the body. This is best achieved by multi-mineral tablet supplements. Spring water and mixed vegetable juice are good sources of minerals and vitamins respectively, but the balance isn't always right for the body's requirements. A diet of fruit juice alone for an extended period, apart from overacidifying the gut, doesn't contain enough of these vital minerals. Some people on long-term fasts have so altered their bodies' salt balance that they died of heart failure. Again, you must take sensible precautions.

These are the advantages and drawbacks to fasting. You must decide for yourself whether you want to try it. If you do, make sure you are in reasonable health and are not too young (teenage or less) or too old (50 or over). Try one or two days at a time first, with two or three weeks between each fast. *Never* fast for longer than three days without medical supervision.

If you have diabetes, or stomach or duodenal ulcers, or if you are expecting or feeding a baby, all fasting is out. With diabetes, the drop of sugar level in the blood could send you into a coma. With gastric ulcers, the initial increased level of acidity in the gut is likely to produce bleeding, and a ruptured ulcer can lead to infected inflammation (*peritonitis*). An expectant or nursing mother on a fast would deprive her baby of essential nutrition, with the possibility of causing damage to the child.

Teenage girls who fast will have an increased tendency to *anorexia nervosa*, the psychological disorder where they cannot face or keep down food at all, even if they want to. Fasting, therefore, is not to be recommended for young women in their teens or early twenties. Fasting is not good, in fact, for any teenagers, since this is a period of growth and development for the body. Girls have the added factor of monthly blood loss sapping their strength. Weight reduction should be achieved by decreasing food intake or changing to a lower-calorie diet and increasing exercise (unless you have to lose weight rapidly under medical supervision). Psychological and physical factors probably both play a part in the onset of *anorexia nervosa*: the condition is hard to reverse and may ultimately have fatal consequences if not checked. It may be caused, therefore, by emotional disturbance, but it is often due to an obsession with weight loss, and usually follows a period of strict (and often unnecessary) dieting.

Warning signs for anybody on a fast are headaches and chest pains. If you experience these, stop fasting immediately and gently build up first mineral salts and carbohydrates, then protein and vitamins, with some fats.

THE HIGH-FIBRE DIET

For nearly a century we have known that lack of fibre, or roughage, in our food predisposes us to constipation, piles (*haemorrhoids*) and varicose veins. Yet during this time we have refined our cereals before we eat them by removing this fibre. Their very whiteness was regarded as an indication of their purity.

The aim should be to have at least one bowel action daily, perhaps two or three. Less than this, or straining in excretion, is an indication that you do not have enough fibre in your diet. Three or more bowel actions daily means you have ample fibre in the diet, perhaps too much, if no other pathological condition is present. There are those who claim that one bowel action every two or three days is adequate: the majority of health authorities would disagree with this.

The other objective of a high-fibre diet is to reduce the time that food takes to pass from one end of the system to the other. With a low-fibre diet this is usually three to five days, and occasionally longer. A high fibre intake reduces this to between one and two days, which is considered ideal as by then the gut has apparently extracted all the nutrients it requires. With some food that is difficult to digest, such as sweet corn or tomato pips, you may be able to assess for yourself how long food takes to pass through your body, since undigested food fragments often appear in the faeces.

By producing appetite satisfaction (*satiety*) at a lower level of food intake, and by increasing the efficiency of elimination, increased fibre in the diet will assist a slow reduction in weight. Furthermore, those foods which are high in fibre are generally low in fat and this also helps to reduce weight.

For those not especially concerned with losing weight, increasing the fibre content of the diet can be beneficial to general health. The range of illnesses that are now attributed to inadequate dietary fibre has been extended from those that were known at the turn of the century.

There is considerable evidence that cancer of the colon (the second most lethal form of the disease after cancer of the lung) and indirectly, through maintaining high blood lipid levels, possibly even cancer of the breast; diabetes and obesity; heart disease and other circulatory problems; gallstones and peptic ulcers (gastric in the stomach; duodenal in the intestine); and diverticulitis are all associated with low-fibre eating. When there is insufficient fibre there is a build-up of fat deposition and high circulating cholesterol, fat and sugar levels; nutrients are incompletely absorbed and toxins remain in the body instead of being eliminated. It is difficult to sort out the contribution to disease of each of the causative factors as they are inter-related, but the evidence is now convincing that inadequate roughage in the diet encourages development of these conditions. Perhaps increasing dietary fibre also exerts a beneficial effect on the body by influencing other biochemical systems in which the role of fibre has not yet been established.

One of the foremost proponents in the world of this change in our eating habits is Denis Burkitt, FRS. He reached his conclusions from a study of the increased prevalence of so-called degenerative diseases in the 'civilized' countries, compared with their occurrence amongst 'primitive' natives in Africa. There, intestinal diseases like ulcerative colitis, cancer of the colon, and diverticulitis are almost unknown. Coronary heart disease is also rare in Africa, China and rural India. These are known as degenerative diseases since they involve an internal wearing down of healthy body functions, as opposed to the infective diseases caused by micro-organisms which invade the body from outside, and which still plague the developing countries.

It was in Britain that the current increase-dietary-fibre movement originated, largely as a result of Denis Burkitt's work. More than a century ago, however, a London medical practitioner, Tom Allinson, realized the benefits of bread baked from whole grain, and more recently the scientific evidence on fibre has been made more accessible by Audrey Eyton's excellent books on what she calls 'The F-Plan Diet'. Apart from being highly readable, these books are full of suggestions for ways to increase roughage in appealing and nutritious recipes.

In terms of actual quantities of fibre consumed, it is estimated that the British eat 15 to 20 g each daily and the Americans 25 to 30 g. These are only average figures; your intake may be higher or lower. It is recommended that we should get 30 to 50 g of fibre in our diet each day;

some primitive tribes consume up to three times that quantity (150 g) daily.

From the figures above you will see that it is almost impossible to reach the recommended daily fibre intake in a total count of 2,000 kcal per day unless a significant portion of high-bran cereals and whole-wheat bread is eaten. To supplement this you will also need to eat fruit or fresh vegetables in reasonable quantities each day. In a healthy diet, there is no room for low-nutrient junk food.

Whatever your source of dietary fibre, increasing your total intake will generally promote better health and also assist in slimming, if you are overweight.

By slowing the process of digestion, fibre is believed to increase the overall absorption of nutrients from food. Even with fibre, however, you should exercise moderation. Too much fibre will carry some heavy metals out of the body along with the waste material. In the case of high-fibre diets involving only a moderate intake of these essential nutrients, depletion or deficiency states are not unknown. With a high-fibre diet (50 g or more daily) you would probably find a multi-mineral supplement in tablet form beneficial, as getting the extra minerals from food is not practicable: the quantities required are just too great.

THE STARCH-BLOCKER DIET

Most of the weight we gain in our bodies comes from two nutrients: the carbohydrates and lipids in our diet. The proteins we eat make muscle tissue but contribute only a little to our calorie count. Our energy comes more or less equally from these other two sources. If we could turn one of them off, we would have a method of eliminating the weight we would otherwise put on as flab.

That is the principle behind the starch-blocker diet. Starch-blockers are pills that are taken to prevent starch being digested, and the resulting glucose absorbed or converted into fat by the body. The chemical name for starch is *amylose* and the enzyme that chops up these polymer molecules, eventually liberating the constituent glucose units, is called *amylase*.

The starch-blocker pill is an extract of raw kidney beans which contains an amylase inhibitor. It was discovered and developed by J. J. Marshall in the US during the 1970s, though the chemical effect has been known for fifty years. It prevents starch being broken down in the gut, but has no action on proteins, lipids or even any other carbohydrates like sugar.

If you don't get your energy from glucose, much of which comes in turn from starch, then your body will turn to the fatty tissue for its energy supply. So on a low-starch diet you lose weight.

Advocates of this approach claim that starch-blocker pills have no side effects, though there hasn't been time yet to evaluate any possible long-term effects. Certainly, in taking these pills, you are tampering with a completely natural and wholly desirable piece of body biochemistry. It is not at all like taking a pill to alleviate symptoms when something has gone wrong.

Some women compare it with taking a daily oral contraceptive pill. If they do that, they say, why not take a starch-blocker pill? In fact, the oral contraceptives interfere as little as possible with body biochemistry. They do prevent ovulation, but this happens every time you're pregnant anyway. They do allow you to have normal periods. Starch-blockers turn off your body's principal energy supply.

Another drawback is that you may get enough glucose for energy from other carbohydrates in your diet – ordinary granulated sugar, lactose from milk, fructose from fruit – and also from ingested lipids, without ever touching your reserve fat supply. Typically, you are likely to get about 100 g of fructose each day (from fruit and that derived from sucrose), and 600 ml (1 pint) milk contains about 25 g of lactose. So there are plenty of alternative sources of glucose apart from starch.

Furthermore, there is an enzyme in saliva called *ptyalin*, which itself breaks down starch into *maltose* (double glucose units) as food is chewed. We secrete at least a litre (1¾ pints) of saliva each day and that contains a lot of ptyalin. Some of the starch you eat will therefore be broken down already before it ever reaches the starch-blockers in your gut.

Even the starch-blocker enthusiasts admit that this treatment is not a complete solution. Certainly it is not an excuse to gorge pasta, chips and every other possible starch source without gaining weight. You still have to modify your eating habits, which brings us back to square one.

Caution

If you do want to try this approach to slimming, make sure you get the proper tablets from a health supplies store. Under no circumstances should you try a do-it-yourself home preparation of starch-blockers. Raw kidney beans contain *haemagglutinins*, which interfere with the oxygen-carrying power of the blood. If you eat raw beans, or take a concoction prepared from them, at the very least you will suffer gastroenteritis, possibly death. Kidney beans should be soaked overnight, boiled vigorously for ten minutes, and simmered for another fifty minutes before they are eaten. By this time, all the amylase blocker is denatured as well as the haemagglutinins.

THE SCARSDALE MEDICAL DIET

This scheme was devised in the 1970s by Dr H. Tarnower, a heart specialist at the Scarsdale Medical Center in New York. The diet involves a tripling of the normal daily protein intake with a great reduction in the calorie-generating foods: carbohydrates are cut by some 10 per cent; lipids are almost halved. The aim is to reduce weight rapidly – up to 9 kg (20 lb) in fourteen days – and to establish healthy eating practices.

The strict diet is followed for only two weeks at a time. In the presence of such a low intake of the normal energy-producing foods, the body will tend to burn off its own resources of fat with the production of chemicals called *ketones*. In the short term the body can cope with this without difficulty, but in the long term it is possible that a toxic state known as *ketosis* could develop. This is why the diet is followed for only two weeks at a time. If you need to lose still more weight, you should come off the diet for at least another fortnight and then go back on it.

The weight loss is achieved by cutting out a number of high-calorie foods:

1 No alcohol.
2 No butter or margarine, even on the two slices of bread allowed daily.
3 No whole milk or cream, or full-fat cheese.
4 No sugar or sweets of any kind, even as desserts.
5 No cakes or biscuits.
6 No potatoes or pasta of any kind.

Apart from the ban on milk and potatoes, most authorities would agree that all the restrictions are beneficial to health, irrespective of weight gain.

The Scarsdale Medical Diet will almost certainly prove effective as a means of weight loss, since the calorie intake from fats and carbohydrates is so low. There are, however, problems which its followers may encounter:

1 It is stressed that the foods laid down in the regimen should be followed without substitutions for each fortnight the diet is pursued. I think many people would find these somewhat restrictive, though there are alternative schemes for vegetarians, gourmets, those needing a low-cost diet, etc.
2 I would be surprised if you were able to get enough fibre in the diet, even though you can eat salads and vegetables almost without limit. With no high-bran cereals, and only two slices of wholemeal bread per day, adequate fibre intake is difficult. Although it is not stated as such,

the implication is that one should use laxatives such as senna or liquorice if there is any problem in bowel movements.

3   You would have to be sure of plenty of variation in the salad, fruit and vegetable ingredients, both for adequate nutrition and to avoid monotony. This variety is not available in many locations at some times of the year.

4   Many people would find taking tea and coffee without either milk or sugar, and bread without butter or margarine, difficult. Diet colas are allowed – but these are high in caffeine and 'additives'.

In other respects the diet provides a far more balanced intake of nutrients than most. With the range of foods offered, provided these are available, there should never be the feelings of hunger or fatigue that so many other diets provoke, nor should you find your diet monotonous. The important issue is whether you enjoy the food. It is extremely difficult to stick to any eating plan which you find tedious, unpleasant or impracticable.

THE MONO-DIET

This term embraces a variety of diets based more or less exclusively on one food.

The milk diet

The milk diet demands drinking only milk (and water). Milk is a highly nutritious food, containing proteins, carbohydrates and lipids and a number of minerals and vitamins – particularly calcium, potassium and phosphorus, and vitamins A and D.

Pasteurization does little to lower the nutritional value of milk and it is necessary to destroy harmful bacteria. In the process, a little vitamin C is lost, but milk is a poor source of this vitamin in any case.

Skimmed milk is a reasonably nutritious food and has many of the nutrients of full milk except for (largely saturated) fats and vitamins A and D. The protein, potassium and calcium content is undiminished.

The main disadvantages of a milk diet are that it fails to provide roughage for elimination; there are not many of the B vitamins or vitamin C in milk; and the saturated fat content of full milk may predispose the dieter to the formation of deposits (*plaques*) of fat on the walls of the blood vessels (a condition known as *atherosclerosis*).

Although in the short term milk is a bland food which doesn't tax the digestive system, there is some evidence that in the long term a high milk intake with inadequate roughage predisposes people to inflammation of the lower intestine (*colitis*) and distention of the intestinal wall into small pouches (*diverticulosis*).

Many people, especially Orientals, cannot tolerate milk (or dairy produce) at all because of hypersensitivity to lactose. They, or others with a predisposition to allergy, may become sensitized to the milk proteins on an exclusive milk diet.

The fruit diet

Not only do grape and grapefruit mono-diets fail to provide adequate nutrition but they also shift the body's balance of salts (*electrolytes*). Grapes and grapefruit have a relatively high level of potassium (up to 400 mg per serving) and little sodium. In moderation this is fine; but if you are eating a few kilograms of fruit each day, it tips the electrolyte balance too far. Neither grapes nor grapefruit possess special enzymes to break down body fat, as is sometimes believed. In the short term (three or four days), however, these diets are effective in producing considerable weight loss.

A diet of pineapple or papaya only should not be pursued for more than a day or two at a time. These fruits contain the protein-breaking enzyme *papain* which, if there are no other foods in the diet, will eventually attack the walls of the gut itself. Normally these are protected by a coating (of the glycoprotein *mucin*), but this breaks down on a low-carbohydrate, low-protein diet. Soldiers serving in Malaya and Burma during the Second World War who were forced to eat nothing but pineapples over an extended period developed this condition. Papain does not affect carbohydrates or lipids, so it needs protein to work on. Pineapple and papaya are fine with one of the other high-protein, low-carbohydrate, low-lipid diets.

The main problem with all mono-diets is that they give you too much of one or two components (even if normally these are beneficial nutrients) and not enough of everything else. Furthermore, even if you like milk or grapes at the start, a few days of this sort of regimen is enough to put you off them for quite a while; which would be a pity, since milk and fruit in moderation are highly nutritious.

The beneficial effects of these diets in curing ailments are almost certainly due to the absence of other foods, additives and contaminants, rather than to the presence of any curative ingredients in the diet food itself. They are not to be recommended for more than occasional use, a day or two at a time.

THE HAY DIET AND MACROBIOTICS

No, this doesn't mean you have to graze in the back garden while the family tuck into their three-course Sunday lunch! This diet takes its name from William Howard Hay, who devised it, based on his own researches together with those of Herbert M. Shelton, John H. Kellogg and V. H. Lindlahr, who were late nineteenth- and early twentieth-century nutritionists. Hay published his own book, *Health Via Food*, in 1934.

The diet is recommended by naturopaths for the treatment of those with a sensitive digestive system. Before explaining the Hay Diet, we must look at what happens to the common minerals in our food when it is digested.

One way of classifying foods is on the basis of the dominant salt (*electrolyte*) residue remaining after digestion. These residues always include one of the mineral elements.

Those foods that produce negative ions like chloride, sulphate and phosphate are designated as *acid-forming*. These ions all contain non-metallic elements (chlorine, sulphur and phosphorus) which, when they are combined chemically with oxygen, form acidic oxides. Such ions are found in high concentration in protein foods like meat, poultry, fish, eggs and some nuts (peanuts and walnuts). Bread and cereals are also in this group; so are plums and prunes (see below).

Foods that have a dominance of metal ions like sodium, potassium, calcium or magnesium are called *base-forming*. These metallic elements all combine with oxygen to form basic or alkaline oxides. Vegetables and fruit (which are predominantly carbohydrate), dairy products and almonds belong to this class of foods.

The acids (like *citric* and *malic acids*) which give fruits their sharp taste are completely oxidized during digestion to give carbon dioxide and water. It is only the basic metallic salt which is left and which makes the fruit base-forming in its overall effect on the digestion.

The organic acids in plums, prunes and the Scandinavian cloudberry (*benzoic acid*), and in American cranberries (*quinic acid*), are not metabolized in the body, so the overall reaction of these fruits is acid- not base-forming.

Foods such as sugar, fats and oils are neutral, being neither acid- nor base-forming.

Now we can get back to the Hay Diet. This decrees that acid-forming and base-forming foods should be kept in proper balance in the diet (20 per cent acid-forming; 80 per cent base-forming) and never mixed at the same meal. Hay was quite correct in asserting that proteins require an acid medium for digestion and carbohydrates an alkaline one. As we have seen, however, in the normal digestive process proteins are broken down in the stomach by acidic gastric juice, while carbohydrates are digested partly by alkaline salivary enzymes and partly by intestinal enzymes as the digestive juice becomes progressively more alkaline.

Some amino acids are more soluble in acid solutions, some in neutral and others in alkaline conditions. The walls of the intestine absorb various amino acids out of the part-digested food (*bolus*) as this is moved along by the gut's rhythmic contractions (*peristalsis*).

There is therefore no biochemical basis for this dietary restriction, but many who follow the Hay Diet claim to be free of indigestion, for which it is mainly prescribed. The healthy body has a finely tuned mechanism to adjust for acidity or alkalinity (*pH*) of foods, so for most people the Hay Diet is an unnecessary inconvenience.

Macrobiotics

There is also some correspondence between the idea of acid- and base-forming foods and the classification of foods according to the Chinese philosophical concepts of Yin and Yang. These are considered to be the negative, passive or female element (Yin) and the positive, active, creative or male element (Yang) of our personality. Well-adjusted individuals are deemed to have a balance between Yin and Yang in their character.

That's the personality side of Yin and Yang. In the macrobiotic approach to diet it is maintained that we must balance the Yin and Yang in our food. Yin foods include nuts, fruit and vegetables; Yang foods include meat, cereals and legumes (or pulses: peas, beans, soya and lentils). The macrobiotic principle is that overall one should aim to make cereals take up 50 to 60 per cent of the diet, fresh vegetables 20 to 30 per cent (except the nightshade family – tomato, potato and aubergine – these are too Yin), and beans 10 to 15 per cent. Fruit, nuts and fish are to be eaten in small amounts only (5 per cent), and meat and dairy produce scarcely at all. There is no restriction about mixing Yin and Yang at one meal, but devotees claim that a lack of Yin/Yang balance leads to physical or mental illness.

This is a very simplified account of macrobiotic dietary philosophy. It is much more than a diet regimen and involves psychic parameters as well as physical ones.

THE BEVERLY HILLS DIET

This comes in two varieties: there's the Beverly Hills Diet (BHD) as such, a six-week regimen for weight loss; and the Beverly Hills Lifetime Diet Plan (BHLDP), an eating scheme for six months or so that establishes the 'correct' eating philosophies to maintain weight indefinitely.

The scheme has been developed over the past decade by Judy Mazel in California. It is essentially a complicated version of the Hay Diet, with many refinements. The central idea, however, is that proteins and carbohydrates should not be eaten together *on the same day*, although either can be eaten with lipids. Each day's diet begins with fruit, the enzymes in which are said to assist the digestion of all the food that follows. Consistent fruit eating (there are certain restrictions in your choices) and Conscious Combining of other foods are the cornerstones of the BHD.

The BHD programme demands that the first nine days of diet should be fruit only, in the next nine days carbohydrates and fats are introduced, and on the nineteenth day proteins are brought back into the diet. The sequence is nutritionally sound and is an elaboration of what has been said in previous chapters. Nine days of fruit-only eating, if it doesn't produce gastritis, will certainly achieve weight loss. Reintroduction of proteins into the diet when you have been without them for a significant length of time should always be preceded by carbohydrates to avoid the ammonia toxicity which is produced by the high level of amino-acid-burning enzymes.

During the slimming period the BHD recommends little or no exercise. Judy Mazel feels that the diet regimen is taxing enough, physically and emotionally, without adding a further stress factor. Many nutritionists would disagree with this recommendation. Only by exercise of as many muscle groups as possible during a fast or period of protein starvation will you encourage the body to burn off its own fat reserves or carbohydrates instead of muscle protein. Fat can only be burned aerobically, which demands fairly vigorous exercise daily.

It is with the BHLDP that most conventional nutritionists would encounter problems, and so might you. Whole-grain cereals, as we have seen, are an excellent source of many vitamins and minerals, apart from their protein and fibre content. As cereals are considered in this scheme as carbohydrates and milk as protein, cereals have to be eaten dry or with butter, if they are eaten at all – not a practicable suggestion for everyone. Legumes (peas, beans and lentils) are high in both protein and carbohydrate, so although they are favoured by most health food devotees, they are not encouraged in the BHLDP.

Once you have established your required weight, there is little restriction on fried foods or saturated fats, provided you follow the other dietary requirements. This is something that almost every medical practitioner and nutritionist, orthodox or otherwise, would take issue with.

As the foods in the full BHLDP are so varied, boredom with eating or deficiencies of any nutrients are most unlikely. There are plenty of people around who have lost weight on the BHD scheme, so if that is your objective, those results are already well proven. Only time will tell if the ongoing BHLDP is nutritionally sound overall; it hasn't been going long enough yet to say one way or the other. Even with the high fruit intake, the saturated fat content and low fibre are the more worrying aspects. Also, some people do develop hypersensitivity reactions to a high fruit intake.

The diet prescribes that ideally you should have no sugar, no white-flour products, no salt, no foods with additives and therefore no soft drinks of the diet variety or otherwise; these are recommendations which most nutritionists would endorse.

You will need to get a grasp of the BHD jargon if you are to make any headway: Conscious Combining, Creative Counterpart, Food Formula, Open Human, Precidotes, are just some of the technical terms used by Judy Mazel in her presentation. All of these make the diet seem more complicated perhaps than it really is. Conscious Combining, for example, is essentially avoiding protein/carbohydrate combinations (the basis of the Hay Diet), and selecting the best fruit to assist digestion of meals (though some fruits have no proven digestive enzyme content). Once you have mastered first the jargon and then the eating principles, it may well be as straightforward as any other diet plan.

Apart from the objections raised above, the main difficulty with the scheme would seem to be that, like most diets, it places considerable restrictions on eating habits, here perhaps more than most. You should avoid legumes, eat cereals without milk, eat nuts only at night, not mix protein and carbohydrate foods (no fish and chips; no meat and vegetables), wait two or three hours even between eating different fruits, or fruits and some other food, eat fruit only before proteins or carbohydrates and never after them in that day, avoid all melons except watermelon, eat grapes or watermelon all day if you eat them at all.... These are just some of the dietary recommendations. This is more rigorous and complicated than most diet plans, even if it is nutritious and effective in reducing or maintaining weight. As with the Hay Diet, for most people whose digestive systems are in reasonable shape, such restrictions are simply not necessary.

As a postscript, I must say I do like Judy Mazel's emphasis on the enjoyment of food. Food should be appreciated and savoured for its appearance, its aroma, and its taste. Once you've swallowed it, it's gone; you can't enjoy it again. It's worth taking the time and trouble to make food appealing to the eye, the nose and the palate, so as to make each meal a gastronomic experience. Judy Mazel brings this out well in her books and also emphasizes the importance of chewing. Mastication is the first stage in the body's processing of food. The more you chew, the less you tax your stomach and intestines and the longer you are able to savour your food – and that, after all, should be one of the reasons for eating in the first place.

Overall, with so many less complicated and safer diets available, the Beverly Hills Diet cannot really be recommended. I suspect its appeal lies largely in its use originally by Hollywood film stars!

12

EXERCISE

General considerations

Daily exercise is beneficial to almost everyone. Even those who suffer from chronic diseases like asthma and arthritis or from heart trouble are encouraged to take regular gentle exercise *under medical supervision* as part of a programme for recovery of health.

Half a century ago, in the Depression, many people couldn't get enough to eat, little was known of nutrition, and work was hard – on the shop floor, in the field, or in the home.

Now we know much more about what nutrients the body needs for health, so that many essential components of diet are added to our food: iodine in salt, vitamins in cereals, calcium in white flour. With labour-saving devices in the home and the fruits of the technological revolution in field and factory, many people don't have to work so hard physically at their jobs. Furthermore, a greater proportion of people nowadays are able to enjoy these labour-saving benefits.

The result is that we now have to seek ways of exercising in order to keep our bodies in shape. The body is made to be used, and the old adage 'use it or lose it' applies to our organs and tissues just as much as it does to animal characteristics in evolution.

Exercise doesn't have to be strenuous for all of the people all of the time. If you are fit enough to do vigorous exercise and you enjoy it you'll probably benefit from it. But even the elderly or the overweight will enjoy better health with deep breathing, brisk walking, tensing and flexing of muscles of the limbs, and greater general activity.

Exercise helps keep your weight down, keeps the vital organs in condition, enables you to breathe better, sleep better and think better, gives you a stronger heart, fewer digestive problems and a better sex life. Exercise funnels your energy overall even if it saps it temporarily. You can cope better with sudden demands on the body such as stress from overwork or injury, or the sudden exertion of running for a bus or train, digging the garden or shovelling snow. Overall, you look better and you feel better.

Strengthening the back muscles helps reduce lower-back pain, a common ailment. Strengthening the abdominal muscles keeps the stomach and other internal organs in place and in better working condition, resulting in less indigestion, constipation or flatulence. Developing the arms and legs allows these potentially stronger muscles to take the strain of increased activity and make less demands on the weaker back or abdominal muscles, reducing the possibility of slipped discs or hernias.

Agility exercises improve motor co-ordination for other tasks and tone up the nerve and blood supply to the muscles and organs. This will increase alertness, perception and digestion, and decrease emotional tension and insomnia.

Without exercise the body atrophies. We are all aware of the feeling of weakness when we are confined to bed for any length of time. It isn't just the sickness itself that saps our reserves; the muscles and internal organs are just not used to the demands made on them by movement once we are up and about again.

In a machine, use produces wear and as a result parts may need to be replaced. This does happen occasionally with the human body when joints that have to bear a heavy load, like the hip, wear down from use and lack of lubricant. Unlike purely mechanical devices, however, the human body has a continuous replacement service. There are systems ready to be called upon for tissue replenishment. However inactive we are, these systems will have to be used from time to time. If these demand occasions are too far apart, the service departments may not be in peak condition. They will be at their best if they are kept occupied with moderate but not excessive work the whole time.

Types of exercise

Exercises are often grouped in one of two ways:

1 Isometric exercises are those which keep the muscles the same length but which change the tension in them. We achieve this by applying force against a steady resistance, as in weight training, with expanders, or the Bullworker, or what the Charles Atlas course used to call Dynamic Tension.
2 Isotonic exercises keep the tension or tone of the muscles constant but alter their length. These are exercises involving movement of the limbs at the joints, as in running, jogging or swimming.

The classification of exercise into aerobic and anaerobic is easy to do in theory but difficult to define in practice.

1 Aerobic exercises are those which increase the pulse and breathing rate. Most of the agility exercises, like prolonged running or jogging, are of this type. Keep-fit classes are an excellent way of combining fitness with social contact, provided they are run by qualified teachers. There are many that have sprung up in recent years that are run by people who do not have the necessary background knowledge of anatomy and physiology.

2 **Anaerobic exercises** mean literally those without oxygen – the sort of exercises which involve great exertion but don't set you panting. Yoga and weight training fall into this category: either very gentle or very short-lived strenuous exercises. Some confusion arises here because exercises which are anaerobic for a person who is fit may be aerobic for one who is unhealthy. You must judge for yourself whether the exercises you do set you panting and make your pulse race.

Anaerobic exercise cannot use lipids as an energy source, only glucose. You need to do extended aerobic exercise to burn off fat. Remember, however, that there is always some oxygen in your tissues so you will always be burning some fat, whatever the exercise, although anaerobic exercise will not burn off enough fat to significantly reduce weight.

Aims of exercise

The resting pulse rate varies between 60 and 90 beats per minute. With sedentary people the pulse rate is generally at the upper end of the range while with athletes it's at the lower end. People who are exceptionally fit may have a pulse rate even lower than 60 beats per minute (*bradycardia*). In general, the fitter you are the lower your pulse rate, though pulse rate also decreases as we grow older. It is always higher in children than in the elderly, irrespective of fitness. This is one of the features of basal metabolic rate that declines with age.

Our pulse rate can double or even treble when we're excited or when we exert ourselves strenuously. A greatly increased pulse rate is also one of the symptoms of shock; again, it can more than double that of the person's resting state (*tachycardia*).

In children and adolescents the heart rate sometimes increases slightly as they breathe in and decreases again as they exhale. This condition (*sinus arrythmia*) is perfectly normal and is no cause for worry. Palpitations or irregularity of the heart beat (*cardiac arrythmia*) under stress or the effects of drugs (including tea or coffee) are also quite normal. If palpitations are not directly attributable to these causes or if they are associated with pain you should seek medical advice.

The normal relaxed breathing rate is about fifteen times per minute. People who are unfit tend to pant with fast short breaths.

Exercise aims to lower the pulse rate, to fill the depths of the lungs by slowing the breathing rate, and to help regularize heart rhythm. This means your heart will have less work to do. Most studies have concluded that deposition of fatty plaques in the blood vessels (*arteriosclerosis*) is less prevalent with a lower heart rate, though some researchers have suggested just the reverse.

Another physiological objective of exercise is to lower blood pressure. The ideal textbook value is 120/60 mm, but anything up to 140/80 is fine. The higher number (*systolic pressure*) is a measure of the pumping strength of the heart. It is increased by emotional stress or exercise. The lower value (*diastolic pressure*) is an indication of the ability of the heart to rest between beats. It is more constant in any one individual and doesn't show the sort of irregularities seen in the upper reading.

Exercise also increases the bulk of muscle tissue: anaerobic exercise is much more effective at doing this than aerobic exercise. Muscles always increase in size with use, including heart muscle. The heart of an athlete, for example, is larger than that of an office worker of equal build, so an enlarged heart is not necessarily a sign of ill health.

Exercise is not always used simply as a means of losing weight overall. The aim is to improve fitness and health, and to convert slack fatty tissue into firm muscle.

It is important that we maintain our bodies at the correct weight. Too much weight, which is the usual problem, means that the vital organs, and especially the heart, have to support a greater tissue mass than is necessary for survival – this means we are overtaxing the sysem. If we have significantly too little weight – and we are not talking here about the odd half kilogram below the ideal weight – then the body has insufficient reserves to cope with the stress of illness, injury, shock, cold, or high workload. Gaining or losing weight is another reason for exercising.

Fitness is measured by mental alertness, physical strength, stamina or endurance, and suppleness of the joints. Internal organs and blood vessels as well as muscles need to stay flexible and supple, maintaining what Dr Donald McLaren called Body Tone. We need this flexibility in the muscles of the heart and gut just as we need it in those of our limbs. Practising yoga is one of the best ways of maintaining suppleness of the limbs and organs.

Practical considerations

If you want to begin an exercise routine you may find the companionship of a sports club or the competition against others in a group an advantage. Companionship also helps if you're out jogging or trying to lose weight.

If you are unfit or unhealthy or overweight, under no circumstances should you embark on a programme of vigorous exercise. Exercises should always be approached gently – with enthusiasm but with control! Throwing your limbs around with abandon can damage muscles, *tendons* (which anchor muscles to bones) and *ligaments* (which bind the bones together at the joints). Again, yoga provides an excellent gentle introduction to an exercise routine.

Try to set aside a regular time for exercise if you can, though many people with a busy schedule find this difficult. Some people enjoy exercise as soon as they get up in the mornings; but others find they need time to let their system wake up properly before they undertake anything so strenuous. Before lunch or before dinner is probably the best time if you can fit this into your daily schedule. Evening exercise before bed is not generally to be recommended because, unless it is really demanding, it is more likely to arouse than relax you.

When you begin, set yourself a goal: to be able to run once around the block without stopping, to do twenty-five push-ups, to run a mile in ten minutes, or whatever. Push the body *just a little* beyond tiredness, but *never* to exhaustion. Never allow yourself to get to the point where muscles are painful or cramped, or you are gasping for air (panting, yes, but *not* gasping).

There are many excellent books on the market now (see Further Reading, page 190) which will give you complete programmes of aerobic and anaerobic exercises with explicit photographs. Some programmes come in the form of cassettes or records with explanatory booklets, so you have a wide choice available.

13

ENERGY

When food is broken down by digestion, some of the constituents are used immediately to build up components needed in the body, and the indigestible part provides roughage. The rest of the metabolic products provide energy: some as heat to keep the body warm; some for doing work; and some to be stored for use later. Of the energy contained in our food, roughly one-third is stored for work and the remaining two-thirds are converted into heat to maintain our body temperature.

Heat energy

The heat supply keeps our bodies at a more or less constant temperature of 37°C (98.6°F), within a range of about 2°F. The body temperature is lowest in the morning and highest in the evening. For women, the lowest (*basal*) body temperature drops to near 36°C (97°F) just before ovulation, ideally in mid-cycle, and rises by some 2°F in the next two or three days before settling down again. Heat energy is retained within our body by the layer of fat under the skin.

Energy for work

When we use muscles to move our limbs during conscious physical activity we are using energy to do work. We also require energy for involuntary movements: our heart must be kept beating and breathing maintained; food and drink must be processed by contractions of the walls of the stomach and intestine; and waste material must be pushed out through the gut and kidneys.

Apart from these physical movements, there are chemical reactions going on in our bodies all the time to process our food, to build or repair tissue, or to store energy. The sending of messages from our sense organs of taste, smell, touch or hearing along the nervous system to the brain involves chemical reactions; so does the detection of light at the back of the eye, enabling us to see as well as sending the message received to the brain. Touch and hearing are physical processes, but taste and smell probably involve chemical reactions as well.

The involuntary physical and chemical processes must continue day and night, whether we are working or resting. This fundamental life-support activity, the basic work the body has to do just to stay alive, in a completely resting state, is known as *basal metabolism*. The speed of our pulse, breathing, and biochemical reactions when we are at rest is called the *basal metabolic rate* (BMR). The BMR is measured at rest; the metabolic rate falls still further during sleep. As we may go for twelve hours or more overnight without food, we need a store of energy we can call on to maintain these processes.

Energy storage

The energy required for biochemical reactions is provided mainly by a molecule called, in shorthand, ATP (*adenosine triphosphate*). The role of ATP in energy exchanges in the body was first suggested as recently as 1941 (by Lipmann and Kalckar). Since then, a number of other energy carriers (*chemotrophs*) have been found. They work in the following way.

When energy is provided by food, it is used to join phosphate groups on to certain organic compounds. The resulting phosphates serve as chemical storehouses of energy. They are said to contain 'energy-rich' phosphate groups because they will liberate their stored energy (a comparatively large amount of energy in chemical terms) when the phosphate groups are split off again. This released energy is then used as described above to provide heat and work.

Some energy carriers liberate more energy than ATP molecules when they shed their phosphate groups. Others release less energy than ATP. This fact is important biologically. As ATP is so widespread in the body, it must have phosphate groups of intermediate potential energy value if it is to function as the principal carrier of energy and phosphate groups from one biological system to another.

Sources of energy

We can get the energy our bodies need to keep warm and to do work by burning food. There are no flames, but the reaction is burning (*combustion*) nonetheless. The energy content of the food we start with is higher than that of the products we end up with, and the energy difference is released and used.

There are two main groups of energy-providing nutrients: carbohydrates and lipids. Each group supplies about 45 per cent of our energy needs; proteins give us the other 10 per cent. Water, vitamins and minerals do not provide us with any energy. The burning of lipids requires the presence of oxygen and is known as *aerobic oxidation*; carbohydrates, on the other hand, can be burned without oxygen so the process is called *anaerobic oxidation*. We obtain more than twice as much energy from the burning of lipids (9 kcal/g) as we do from the same weight of proteins or carbohydrates (4 kcal/g).

One way to turn on our energy-burning reactions is by exercise. Another way is by stimulation of the nervous system. How well we get through the day is often a matter of energy supply. We may eat because we are hungry or out of habit, but we drink extra cups of tea or coffee (more than we need to quench our thirst), or take glasses of sherry or smoke cigarettes because we need an additional lift. The nutritional value of a cup of coffee or even a glass of sherry is small. The nutritional value of a cigarette is nil. The reason we want them is to give a stimulus to the nervous system to pour out more adrenaline. This, in turn, makes the liver and muscles break down more glycogen. Any extra carbohydrate boosts the blood sugar further and we get still more energy.

Energy from the sun

We have looked at how the body uses energy, how it is stored, and where we get energy from in our food. But where does all this energy originate from in the first place? It's one of the fundamental laws of physics that we cannot create or destroy energy, so our food sources must get their energy from somewhere.

All the energy we derive from our food comes originally from the sun. Plants use sunlight, together with *chlorophyll*, to convert carbon dioxide and water into carbohydrates – starch (for their food supply) and cellulose (for their structural tissue). This is the reverse of the reaction that we carry out in our bodies to liberate that energy when we burn carbohydrates. Under ordinary conditions in the laboratory, carbon dioxide would simply dissolve slightly in water to form carbonic acid. It is the presence of the sunlight and chlorophyll which builds up carbon dioxide and water vapour molecules into the larger organic molecules we call carbohydrates. This process is known as *photosynthesis*.

Animals which chew the cud convert the grass they eat into their tissue protein; so when we eat meat for energy even this is derived from grass which has grown under the action of sunlight.

In the sea, plants use carbon dioxide together with dissolved mineral salts to build their carbohydrate tissues in the presence of sunlight. Fish eat the tiny floating plants and animals called *plankton*, which themselves have derived their growth energy from the sun.

So whether we eat meat, fish, or vegetation for our food energy, the original source of that energy is the sun.

Reaction energy – the role of enzymes

One of the reasons we need energy from food is to power our bodies' chemical reactions. Some of these reactions give out energy when they occur (*exothermic reactions*), while others take in energy (*endothermic reactions*). Whether energy is given out or taken in overall as a result of a reaction, chemicals need an energetic push, called the *activation energy*, if they are to react together in the first place. The molecules have to climb over an energy barrier so that they can get close enough to each other to react. Enzymes make these reactions occur more quickly or more slowly, or make them happen at a lower temperature (the body temperture), by lowering or raising this energy barrier.

The body has two sets of tissue-processing reactions, both of which are going on all the time, day and night. There are building-up processes (*anabolism*) and wearing-down processes (*catabolism*), and some of the reactions will generate energy while others use it up.

Energy input

The amount of energy we put into our bodies depends on two factors: what we eat and how much we eat. As we have seen, every gram of protein or carbohydrate generates 4 kcal of energy and every gram of fat produces 9 kcal of energy. In total, we need about 2,000 to 3,000 kcal per day (or about 10 MJ/day).

The energy distribution amongst our daily food intake is roughly as shown in Table 4. This illustrates also the different energy values of different types of food. Naturally, the exact proportions will vary from one individual to another, but the table gives an approximate idea of where the energy comes from.

Table 4   Food energy sources in the average daily diet

	kcal
80 g (2¾ oz) of protein	320
80 g (2¾ oz) of lipid	720
340 g (12 oz) of carbohydrate	1,360
Total energy provided	2,400

This is based on an average energy allowance of 2,400 kcal per day. In the first six years of life children need under 2,000 kcal daily; adolescent boys may need 3,000 kcal or more; men doing manual labouring may require 3,500 to 4,000 kcal each day; and really strenuous activity can demand in excess of 5,000 kcal daily. You can adjust the figures in Table 4 as appropriate for your own needs and diet.

Let's take a look now at how specific diet items make up these totals for protein, lipid and carbohydrate. Table 5 shows the breakdown for a

Table 5   Distribution of proteins, lipids and carbohydrates amongst the food in a typical day's menu

Food	Protein (g)	Lipid (g)	Carbohydrate (g)
Breakfast:			
600 ml (1 pint) whole milk (with cereal and tea/coffee)	20	20	30
2 shredded wheat biscuits *or* 50 g (1¾ oz) wheat flakes	4		40
4 teaspoons sugar (with cereal and tea/coffee)			20
2 slices bread (white or wholemeal)	5		30
butter		8	
Midday meal:			
90 g (3 oz) full-fat cheese	20	30	
2 slices bread (white or wholemeal)	5		30
mixed salad			20
butter		8	
1 slice cake		6	50
2 teaspoons sugar (with tea/coffee)			10
Evening meal:			
115 g (4 oz) lean beef steak (or 90 g/3 oz tuna in brine) (or two-egg omelette)	36 (24) (10)	8	
90 g (3 oz) peas and 90 g (3 oz) carrots			15
1 large potato	3		60
fruit salad			25
2 teaspoons sugar (with tea/coffee)			10
Totals:	80 (mean) (min. 67, max. 93)	80	340

typical day's menu, and also indicates how the quantity and quality of the food we eat affect energy input.

Energy output

Just as there are two factors which affect weight gain, there are also two factors which determine weight loss – the energy we use up. The first of these is the basal metabolic rate, and the second is the amount of conscious exercise we take. We have enormous energy reserves within the body: for example, 1,000 kcal are stored as carbohydrates; 24,000 kcal are stored as proteins; and 141,000 kcal are stored as lipids.

If we want to lose weight, it's much easier to eat less food or less energy-rich food than to try to burn off the excess by exercise. The current textbooks generally have it that 1 kg weight is equivalent to 9,000 kcal (38,000 kJ), or 1 lb is equivalent to 4,100 kcal (17,000 kJ). That much energy represents a great deal of exercise, as we shall see later.

It is worth pointing out that these are the most pessimistic figures for weight/energy equivalents. They are based on the assumption that all the weight lost is fat (at 9 kcal/g). In practice, this will not be so. When fatty (*adipose*) tissue is broken down, some of the stored carbohydrates and water will go too. Water has no calorific value and carbohydrates have a greater weight equivalent per calorie than fats. Therefore, you may be able to lose 0.5 kg (1 lb) with as little as 2,000 kcal (or 8,000 kJ) of exercise.

Basal metabolic rate: this is our involuntary energy output. The BMR depends on several factors:

1 Our body size. The bigger we are, the greater the surface area of skin, and hence the greater heat loss.
2 Our weight. The greater the thickness of the fat layer covering the body, the better the insulation, and the lower the heat loss.
3 Our state of health. Many diseases are accompanied by fever in which we lose more heat than usual from our bodies, and the BMR is raised. However, malnutrition is accompanied by a lowering of the BMR. Fasting produces a similar lowering in rate after three to four days.
4 Our genetic make-up. The endocrine glands determine the rates of our biochemical reactions. It is the secretions of the thyroid, and adrenaline from the adrenal glands that do most to speed up the body's chemistry. Also, the hormones from the sex glands govern our sexual desire and activity, and indirectly this stimulates another energy output.
5 Our age. While we are growing, our BMR steadily increases, both because of the growth activity and because of the increase in body size.

73

Table 6   Energy output of a 64 kg (10 stone) male office worker and of a 57 kg (9 stone) housewife with children

Man	kcal/day
8 hours sleeping	510
6 hours sitting (reading, writing, watching TV, commuting)	480
1 hour walking (around office and commuting)	190
5 hours office activity	730
2½ hours eating meals	190
1 hour general activities (walking up and down stairs, playing with children)	220
½ hour personal preparation (showering, shaving, dressing)	80
Total:	2,400

Woman	kcal/day
8 hours sleeping	460
4 hours sitting (reading, writing, sewing, knitting, watching TV)	290
4 hours standing (shopping, cooking)	275
2 hours walking	345
2½ hours eating meals	170
1 hour playing with children	200
2 hours housework (ironing, cleaning, laundry, making beds)	400
½ hour personal preparation (showering, hair washing, dressing)	70
Total:	2,210

Based on data originally quoted in *Physiological Measurements of Metabolic Functions in Men* by C. F. Consolazio, R. E. Johnson and L. J. Pecora, McGraw-Hill, 1963.

After maturity it slowly declines into old age. This decrease in BMR after middle age (menopause) is one of the factors contributing to the weight increase often experienced at this time, if food is not cut back or an exercise programme maintained.

Table 7 Energy output of a 64 kg (10 stone) adult in various sporting activities

	kcal/hour
walking (3 mph on level ground)	215
calisthenics	260
cycling	265
playing tennis	365
swimming	522
playing squash	550
running (7 mph on level ground)	740

Based on data originally quoted in *Physiological Measurements of Metabolic Functions in Men* by C. F. Consolazio, R. E. Johnson and L. J. Pecora, McGraw-Hill, 1963.

Activity: this is our voluntary energy output. We use up energy in everyday activities whether we take deliberate exercise or not. Table 6 gives a general idea of the amount of energy used up in household chores or work in an office, and Table 7 gives typical energy values of some sporting activities.

To some extent the personality factor is determined for us. We have an inherent tendency to be active or passive, to be bright and cheerful or sad and melancholic, to be positive or negative in our outlook. Of course, at one time or another in our lives we will probably all show all of these personality traits, but we all tend towards one pole of behaviour or the other.

Superimposed on the basic personality tendency that we are born with is the personality that we develop for ourselves, determined by our experience of life. We decide for ourselves that we need more exercise if we lead a sedentary life; we may opt for a vigorous and energy-consuming social life; we resolve to take things a little easier in our working day as we move into middle or old age; and so on. All of this affects our voluntary energy expenditure and our BMR.

The energy equation

We have seen that there are two things which determine how much weight we put on (what we eat and how much we eat), and two things which govern what weight we burn up in energy (the basal metabolic rate and activity).

Whether we want to gain or lose weight, or just stay healthy at our present weight, we have to balance these amounts of energy (see Figure 4).

This idea of monitoring body weight without tiresome calorie counting is something we shall now go on to explore in detail in the next chapter.

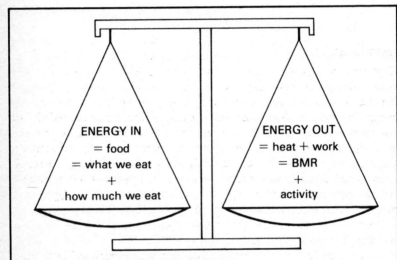

ENERGY IN
= food
= what we eat
+
how much we eat

ENERGY OUT
= heat + work
= BMR
+
activity

Figure 4   Balancing the energy equation

Note   The term 'work' on the right-hand side of the scales includes work done during exertion as well as the involuntary movements of the heart, lungs and chemicals around the body.

14

THE GOOD-HEALTH PLAN

Introduction

Anybody can lose (or gain) weight, whatever their eating or activity habits are now, if they really want to change (and provided they have no hormonal disorder). A knowledge of how your body gets and uses its energy supply, and determination to succeed are all that is needed: but you cannot achieve your goal without these. If the mental effort put into crash dieting or exercising were spent on *balancing* eating and activity, there would not be so many frustrated dieters or fatigued joggers around.

In a crash diet you will indeed lose weight, but you may lose most of it first as carbohydrate, then as protein. Once you start eating again you may well replace lost lean muscle tissue (protein) with flab (lipid).

Eating whatever you want and frantically exercising to keep the weight off is no solution either. The foods you eat may contribute to flab rather than nutrition, and exercise will then tax an undernourished body.

Neither diet nor exercise alone is the answer. Whatever the diet books say and whatever the exercise books imply, there is only *one* route to persistent health and fitness. If you have stayed with me thus far you will know by now that you *must* combine the two: sensible eating with regular activity. You need a sensible but nourishing and enjoyable selection of food that you can live with for the rest of your life without anxiety or boredom. With that you need a pace of life, an exercise routine, an activity attitude which will burn off enough calories to keep pace with your food intake.

If, for some reason, you are forced to eat richer food for a while, you must cut back on other foods or take more exercise, or both. If pressure of work cuts out some of your exercise time, cut out some of the calorie-rich foods as well. If you don't adjust the food/activity, energy-in/energy-out relation, you will gain or lose weight. As many people know to their chagrin, it is so much easier to put it on than take it off.

You should not look on this as something negative. Take any extra exercise you need as hiking, swimming, tennis or dancing, and *enjoy* it. Change to *exciting* low-calorie foods: there are plenty of them about and many books to tell you how to prepare them in an appetizing way. There is no need to subject yourself to tedious food and torturous exercise. It is only by choosing food and exercise you enjoy that you will be able to live with any restrictions they might impose.

I have summarized the main recommendations in the section at the end of this chapter.

How to set about achieving your weight goal

The preceding chapters give you the information you need to work out the energy balance in your own case.

First, you need to monitor your weight by weighing yourself without clothes, using the same scales, first thing each morning before you start eating. Some people weigh a few kilograms more at night than in the morning. The difference is accounted for by sweating, urination, defecation and basal metabolism over the ten- to twelve-hour period between supper and breakfast. It's important, too, to be completely naked for the weigh-in each time: it's tempting to persuade yourself that a single item of underwear really does weigh a couple of kilograms!

Now you need to decide whether your weight needs to go up, down, or stay the same.

Weight and build

If you want to know whether or not you are the ideal weight, consult Table 8. The weights indicated here are for a person of medium build. By 'build' we mean thickness of bones and bulk of supporting muscle tissue. If you are of heavy build, *add* 4 kg (8 lb) to the bottom of the range and 5 kg (10 lb) to the top. If you are of light build, *subtract* 3 kg (6 lb) from the bottom of the range and 4 kg (8 lb) from the top.

It is very easy to be genuinely mistaken or to cheat just a little bit in assessing which type of build you are, but the wide ranges of weight for each height give you quite a lot of latitude for error.

One further point: fashions change, and women, particularly, may sometimes be considered more fashionable when they are lean and slender or sometimes when they are well endowed. The result is that whatever weight is considered 'normal' in a population will change from one time to another. There is also considerable racial variation: American negroes and Polynesians are often large-framed, while Indians and Japanese tend to be small-built, so normal weight ranges will also change from place to place. This is why no two sets of weight tables are ever likely to give you precisely the same ranges. Depending on how widely you read, they may well differ by a few kilograms in what is considered 'ideal'. So the tables given here should be taken only as a guide. A couple of kilograms astray either way are of no consequence if you can see for yourself that you are adequately covered with firm tissue.

Table 8 Ideal weight ranges for men and women of medium build

| MEN | | | | | WOMEN | | | | |
| Height | | | Ideal weight range | | Height | | | Ideal weight range | |
cm	ft	in	kg	lb	cm	ft	in	kg	lb
198	6	6	81-91	178-200	183	6	0	67-76	148-167
196	6	5	79-89	174-196	180	5	11	65-74	143-163
193	6	4	77-87	169-191	178	5	10	63-72	139-159
191	6	3	75-85	165-187	175	5	9	61-70	134-154
188	6	2	72-82	159-181	173	5	8	60-68	132-150
185	6	1	70-80	154-176	170	5	7	58-67	127-148
183	6	0	68-78	150-171	168	5	6	56-65	123-143
180	5	11	66-76	146-167	165	5	5	54-63	119-139
178	5	10	65-73	143-161	163	5	4	52-61	115-134
175	5	9	63-71	139-156	160	5	3	50-59	110-130
173	5	8	61-69	134-152	157	5	2	49-57	108-125
170	5	7	59-67	130-148	155	5	1	48-55	105-121
168	5	6	57-65	125-143	152	5	0	46-54	101-119
165	5	5	55-63	121-139	150	4	11	45-52	99-115
163	5	4	53-61	117-134	147	4	10	44-51	97-112
160	5	3	51-59	112-130	145	4	9	42-50	93-110
157	5	2	50-58	110-127	142	4	8	41-49	90-108
155	5	1	49-57	108-125					
152	5	0	47-55	103-121					

Physique is a far better guide than weight to tell you whether you are in condition.

One of the best ways of judging your weight, apart from the scales, is to stand naked in front of a full-length mirror. If bones are distending your skin all over the place, you may need to gain a little weight. You probably feel the cold easily and get tired quickly as well. If, on the other hand, there are rolls of flab (as opposed to a layer of firm fat) around your jowls, hips, the upper parts of your arms and legs, and over your belly and buttocks, you don't need your scales and these weight tables to tell you that you ought to shed a little weight. The size of your breasts accounts for a few kilograms of weight in the case of women, but this is something you can do little about – it is largely (though not entirely) hormonal.

Now that you've decided which way your weight has to go, how do you set about it? Let's consider each method in turn.

How to gain weight

Suppose you are a lean 51 kg (8 stone) 18-year-old male, and you want to train for the Mr Universe competition. At your present weight you will probably need less than 2,000 kcal a day to start. You need to build up slowly over six to twelve months to 3,500 or 4,000 kcal per day. If you do highly strenuous activity you may even need 5,000 to 7,000 kcal each day.

You must keep a balance between protein, carbohydrate and lipid, with plenty of vitamins and minerals, but high on the protein (100 to 140 g daily): lean meat, poultry, fish, nuts and avocado.

Lipids should be unsaturated fats as far as possible. On no account should you stuff yourself with rich food and sweets; these put on weight of the wrong kind. Dairy produce is acceptable in moderation, but not more than just over a litre (2 pints) of whole milk daily (800 kcal), or the equivalent in full-fat cheese and butter, even on a 4,000 kcal diet.

Carbohydrates come from cereals, fruit and vegetables. You'll need to go easy on the salads and cottage cheese – as these will fill you up with water and not provide enough nutrient or roughage for their weight.

Through all of this you need constant exercise, making sure you work as many groups of the body's muscles as possible in each session. You'll need at least one hour of vigorous exercise daily, aerobic and anaerobic, but you can take this in two half-hour sessions or three of twenty minutes each. A little exercise taken regularly is better than trying a long, demanding session, especially when you start.

How to lose weight

If you are considerably overweight, you should consult your family doctor before embarking on any diet to make sure that your condition is not the result of diabetes or endocrine disorder. If this should be the case, you may need drugs to supplement your diet. If you are in reasonable health but simply a little overweight, by following the sensible eating suggestions given here you should lose weight without the need for any fad or crash diets.

If you want to reduce weight, it's always better to do this gradually if you can, preferably no more than 1 kg (2¼ lb) per week. This allows your body to re-adjust its metabolism slowly with the least effect on your vital organs. Faster weight loss may seem psychologically uplifting, but it is more likely to produce fatigue and depression, both of which are frequent but perfectly normal symptoms if you lose a lot of weight quickly.

One kilogram of fat is equivalent to 9,000 kcal or 38,000 kJ; one pound of fat is generally stated to be equivalent to about 4,100 kcal or 17,000 kJ. The figures don't look quite so depressing in Imperial units! This assumes that all your weight loss will be from fat itself, which isn't in fact strictly true (see page 73).

Let's suppose that you are a 30-year-old woman weighing in at 76 to 89 kg (12 to 14 stone) and keen to get back to that sylph-like you of yesteryear. For success and health, without fatigue, irritability or boredom, you will have to accept that reconditioning is a slow process. You have to re-educate your mind as well as your body. Grit and determination for a ten-day crash diet may work wonders by the end of this period, but, as explained in earlier chapters, over the next ten days you're likely to put all the weight back on again, perhaps even replacing some of the firm muscle you had before with flabby fat.

The first priority is to enjoy your diet, your exercise, and your life. This slimming-down is supposed to make a happier and healthier you, so it's no good being miserable about getting there.

First, think of the end-product: the streamlined person who will feel healthier and look more attractive. You won't feel so tired and sluggish, nor will you put as great a strain on your heart if you don't have all that excess weight to carry around.

Based on the energy equation discussed at the end of the last chapter (see page 75), you need to work off *each day* more energy than you put in with your food, so all the food you eat must be nutritious. You cannot afford to do without essential nutrients, so there's no room for junk food. Start by reducing the amount you eat, and as rapidly as possible, cutting out *all* fried foods; poach or grill instead. Potatoes baked in their jackets are fine, even moistened before serving with a *small* pat of butter or a little milk, but all chips, crisps and French fries are out. Bread is nutritious, too, but wholemeal only and not more than two or three slices a day, *scraped* with butter or vegetable oil margarine.

Cereals are highly nutritious, but concentrate on the bran-enriched or whole-grain varieties; once again, the sugar-coated forms are not to be included in your menu. Take cereals with low-fat milk. You'll find there's great variation in the fat content and the taste of 'low-fat' milk, so experiment a little to find the one that suits you, and look at the ingredients. You want skimmed or semi-skimmed milk.

Red meat should be completely avoided because there's quite a lot of (saturated) fat even in the leanest cuts. Concentrate on poultry and fish for your protein; but not mackerel, eels, sardines or tuna in oil (although tuna in brine is allowed). Nuts should be avoided or eaten sparingly. They are high in fibre and protein, but also high in lipids.

Fresh or dried fruit, vegetables and salads are great; eat as much as you can cope with. The water content will help fill you up. They are full of fibre, minerals and vitamins, and will provide you with easily digestible carbohydrate (starch) for energy.

All tinned food, except tuna and salmon, should be eliminated from your diet. Tinned fruit has too much syrup; tinned vegetables have too many preservatives, especially salt; and both fruit and vegetables lose some of their micronutrients in the canning process or with time. All tinned and pre-packed meats should be avoided as they have too much sodium-everything: chloride, nitrate, nitrite, etc.

You will need to minimize and, if possible, eliminate alcohol from the diet. Preferred drinks are tap water, spring or mineral water, herbal tea, dandelion coffee (the last two with the minimum of sugar and only skimmed or semi-skimmed milk), fruit juice, vegetable juice (both drunk sparingly – no more than 250 ml or ½ pint each day).

So much for the food. Now for the exercise. This is more likely to be a chore if you don't think a little about it first. To start off with, choose a gentle activity that you can share with someone, such as a game of golf, or walking, or going to a beginners' keep-fit class. There are plenty of facilities around these days, even in small centres. The social contacts will provide you with the benefit of someone to share your activities with as well as the possibility of making friends.

This sort of activity is likely to be only once or twice a week, however, and that's nowhere near enough exercise. In between times, using any of the exercise workbooks as a guide and some suitable up-tempo music on a cassette or stereo, do your own exercises at home. Make sure you have as few clothes on as possible so you're not restricted, and keep a window open while you work out. You want the maximum air supply you can get.

Jogging in traffic in the centre of a city is *not* to be recommended. You will almost certainly do more harm than good by forcing your lungs to take in extra helpings of carbon monoxide, lead compounds, and numerous other pollutants. No exercise at all must be better than jogging (or cycling strenuously) in traffic.

At the start, the diet plus exercise will be an effort – but isn't everything that's worth doing? After only a few days, at the very least you'll begin to feel more supple; after a week or so, you'll begin to see the difference. But don't expect miracles. This is intended to be a slow process and a long-term food and exercise prescription for health.

The myth of calorie counting

Where, you may be asking, is all the calorie information I need to measure my food intake? Forget it! Calorie counting is a chore. It ruins what should be one of the joys of life: eating. It's difficult to do accurately, and it isn't even necessary.

Why are you counting calories in the first place? Probably to minimize weight gain. Then balance your weight by sensible eating, as outlined here, and monitor your weight with the scales – which you'd do in any case even if you were calorie counting. To weigh out portions of food and take your pocket calculator to dinner is enough to spoil anybody's appetite.

Weigh yourself each morning. Decide whether or not today you can indulge a little. Then relax and enjoy yourself. Do you realize how delicious poached trout or paella with salad or vegetables can be?

How to maintain weight and keep fit

If you're just the right weight and it's a question of staying that way, judicious eating along the guidelines given here with plenty of gentle exercise and a little vigorous activity is the prescription.

Try to exercise each day if you can; but if not, half an hour two or three times a week will suffice, if you push yourself just a little, as long as you're sensible in your selection of food.

Remember, the ideal weight is in the middle of the range with no surplus flab. There are those who advocate that your weight should be as low as possible, at the bottom of the range, but if this is so, you will have no reserves for stress or illness, when you may have an increase in BMR through fever, or loss of weight from sickness, diarrhoea or lack of appetite. This will make the illness more damaging and recovery slower. Once again, the working principle is moderation: aim for the middle of the weight range. You should not aim to be as thin as you can possibly be and still stay alive – because you may not, if you overdo it.

Summary
REDUCE:

Saturated fat
1 Use lean meat, fish and poultry for protein and avoid high-fat meats like bacon, pork, veal, lamb or tongue.
2 Use dairy produce only in moderation, although there is no need to avoid it completely as cream is a good source of vitamins and minerals.
3 Use skimmed (under 1 per cent fat) milk or semi-skimmed (2 per cent fat) milk in preference to silver top (4 per cent fat) milk, and avoid gold top (5 per cent fat) milk.
4 Use lower-fat cheeses like Camembert or Brie, Gouda or Edam (under 25 per cent fat) in preference to high-fat cheeses like Cheddar and Stilton (over 33 per cent fat).

5   Use only four or five eggs a week, remembering the ones you use in cooking.

6   Use tinned tuna in brine instead of oil, or soak up excess oil with kitchen towels.

7   Use poaching or grilling instead of frying.

8   Use safflower, sunflower or corn oils or their margarines, and avoid coconut or palm oil; suet, lard and dripping should be banished from the kitchen.

9   Use satisfying, interesting and nutritious foods at set mealtimes, so that you avoid snack foods between meals.

Sugar

1   Use raw sugar instead of refined white or brown so that you get extra minerals.

2   Use sugar-coated cereals only if mixed with unsweetened cereals.

3   Use fruit for sweetening instead of cane sugar; it's still sugar but it will give you fructose, which is sweeter than sucrose, and fibre, minerals and vitamins as well.

4   Use fruit with bread and butter instead of jams or marmalade; even high-fruit 'extra jams' contain around 70 per cent sugar.

5   Use fresh fruit instead of tinned as tinned fruits usually contain syrup and may have lost much of their nutrient content.

Sodium

1   Use fresh or frozen vegetables; tinned ones have more salt, which is difficult to remove, and fewer nutrients.

2   Use fresh meat, not tinned or packaged meats as these contain sodium chloride and sodium nitrite or nitrate.

3   Use spices or herbs for flavouring instead of salt; or you can even try the real taste of food, without any additives.

Drugs

1   Use herbal teas, dandelion coffee, fruit juice or mineral water instead of tea, coffee or alcohol.

2   Use pharmaceutical drugs *only* when you really need them.

INCREASE:

Fibre, minerals and vitamins

1   Use fresh, raw fruit and fresh vegetables instead of tinned.

2   Use whole-grain bread and cereals, and avoid refined foods with white flour and white rice.

3   Use vitamin and mineral supplements only if they are non-toxic and only if you can be reasonably sure your food intake is inadequate for your needs.

Exercise

1   Take fifteen to thirty minutes' vigorous exercise three or four times a week – enough to make you pant but not gasp.

BALANCE:

1   Sodium input with twice as much potassium; there's no need to avoid salt completely.

2   Saturated fat with at least twice as much unsaturated fat; there's no need to avoid meat, milk, cheese and cream completely.

3   Most importantly: balance energy input from food with energy output from activity.

Remember

Foundations of good or ill health are laid in youth. Start your children on this health plan so they get used to it while they are young. Some children now have no games or gym periods in school because of timetable problems, and have a limited selection of foods available from school dinners. They also have a greater than ever tendency and opportunity to experiment with drugs.

If you are no longer young, you can still extend your life expectancy and years of enjoyment by sensible living.

Once your health plan is established, don't worry about it or an occasional transgression from the ideal objectives you have set yourself. Relax. Enjoy your food and your exercise, and the better health that you will inevitably achieve.

15

SEX

Although ideally an expression of love, sex is also good exercise and one of the best ways of releasing tension. Statistical evidence indicates that middle-aged married men are much less likely to suffer strokes, heart attacks, or commit suicide than single men. Regular, and for the most part probably unspectacular, sexual activity is likely to be a contributing factor.

During sexual activity, especially to orgasm, pulse and breathing rates increase considerably. It thus becomes an aerobic exercise, with all the usual benefits if pursued regularly.

Sex in marriage, though it can and should still be exciting, doesn't carry with it the uncertainty or the need for outstanding performance that usually accompanies casual sexual experience. There is a comfortable reassurance about knowing the needs, desires, and foibles of your partner.

For women, love, emotional and psychological factors play a bigger part in sexual activity and fulfilment than for men. That is not to say that men do not participate emotionally in sex or get anything other than physical release from sexual activity, nor that women do not enjoy the physical aspects of sex. It is just that, biologically, sex is a physical and essential activity for a man, but an emotional and optional activity for a woman, albeit a highly pleasurable and desirable option. Adolescent boys will have spontaneous orgasms and emissions, usually at night (nocturnal emissions or wet-dreams), even if their dreams have no erotic content. Girls rarely experience spontaneous orgasms.

The ability to participate in satisfying sexual activity, provided it is not to excess in either frequency or performance, seems to slow down the ageing process. It also reduces the need for excesses of food, tobacco, alcohol or drugs as a means of releasing tension.

There need be no taboos in sexual activity provided it is what both partners want. There is always tension in a relationship if, in order to provide satisfaction for one, the other is forced to endure pain or humiliation which he or she does not want. It must be said, however, that there are some who enjoy a certain amount of physical pain during sex, and who find it stimulating. The need to inflict pain or to endure it is a regular part of sexual activity for some people. Whatever is mutually acceptable should be permissible.

Masturbation is for some a contentious issue, but the Kinsey and Masters & Johnson studies indicate that it is a widespread and, in that sense, entirely normal sexual practice for both men and women. Indeed, it often forms part of a couple's sexual activity together. For those who do not have a partner, it provides a safe release of sexual tension, and for adolescent boys it avoids nocturnal emissions. It becomes undesirable only if solitary stimulation is preferable to mutual satisfaction and one partner of a couple is left frustrated. The old warnings of the dire physical consequences which resulted from masturbation have no basis in fact and were a hangover of Victorian prudery and repression. Masturbation or manual stimulation is often an effective way of achieving orgasm.

For those who have difficulty in reaching orgasm, concentrating on it and struggling to reach a climax may make it more elusive. It will happen more easily if you think of your partner and his or her caresses, and enjoy the getting there.

Contraception

Of the contraceptive methods available, the daily hormone pill for women is generally regarded as the most reliable and aesthetically satisfactory, as the contraceptive precautions do not have to be taken immediately before the sex act. The pill mimics the biochemistry of the natural ovulatory cycle, but allows monthly bleeding to occur without ovulation. For young women in good health the pill is a safe and reliable method of contraception, with a risk factor smaller even than that of having a baby. There is no convincing evidence that the pill causes cancer of the breast or of the cervix. Some women do experience side effects, the most common being weight gain or weight loss, headaches, and (though most would regard this as a benefit) lighter periods. The pill should not be used by young teenage girls because it may interfere with the growth process, but in the late teens and up to the menopause it is generally accepted as being the most satisfactory method of contraception.

For those who cannot tolerate the pill, or who are heavy smokers, or are approaching the menopause, or who may have a predisposition to circulatory problems, the intra-uterine device (IUD) is a common alternative. This is a physical coil of wire, usually plastic-coated, placed inside the neck of the uterus. It appears to work by creating a biochemical environment in the uterus which prevents implantation of the egg cell. Most women using IUDs experience stomach cramps for the first three or four months, but after this period these should decrease to a negligible level or disappear altogether. If strong abdominal pain persists you should always return to your doctor or family planning clinic. The IUD usually provokes heavier monthly periods and many women find they need an iron supplement (which you should always stop taking at least three or four days before menstrual bleeding begins – see page 174). The IUD is not recommended for women who lead a very active life, especially those who play tennis, squash, or go riding. The jogging of the body can dislodge the device into places where it should not be.

The barrier methods – a condom or sheath for men and a diaphragm cap for women – are simple and reasonably effective, particularly if used with a chemical contraceptive. They have the aesthetic disadvantage of having to be applied just before intercourse takes place. Hypersensitivity reactions to the chemical spermicides are not unknown, but they can often be eliminated by changing to another brand.

So-called 'natural' methods of contraception are notoriously unreliable. Although some couples can make them work satisfactorily, many more have found that they result in unplanned pregnancies.

Whatever your sexual preferences or opportunities, sexual fulfilment makes a beneficial contribution to health, and in a programme of planned eating and exercise it should not be neglected. Unfortunately, satisfying, relaxed or vigorous sex is another health benefit, along with exercise, that tends to get sacrificed to the pressures of modern everyday life.

16
SLEEP

What is sleep?

Before we discuss why we need to sleep and how we can achieve it, it would be helpful to explain how doctors define sleep. Nowadays the state of being asleep is assessed by the electrical activity of the brain, using a machine called an EEG (*electroencephalogram*).

As we fall asleep, there are four stages of progressively increasing unconsciousness. The electrical waves in our brain when we are awake are called *alpha-waves*; they occur with a frequency of 8 to 12 cps or cycles per second (that is, there are between 8 and 12 complete waves occurring in every second).

The first stage of sleep, which lasts for only a few seconds or a few minutes, is indicated by the gradual disappearance of these alpha-waves. The second stage is denoted in the brain wave trace by *spindles* of frequency 13 to 15 cps with occasional *spikes*. There are now more waves per second: the brain has become more active. Stage three is marked by the appearance of longer waves, called *delta-waves*, with a lower frequency of 1 to 4 cps (fewer waves per second: more gentle brain activity). The fourth and final stage of sleep is defined when these delta-waves take over most of the brain wave picture.

This is a more detailed analysis of sleep than we shall need here; we shall use a simpler description. Stages one and two are grouped together and called the *D state* (the dreaming phase). This is characterized by *rapid eye movements*, and for this reason this phase is called REM sleep. Stages three and four are grouped together as the *S state* (for synchronized brain waves).

Physiology of sleep

We do all our dreaming and perhaps some sleep-talking during the D phase. The electrical activity in the brain is quite intense and irregular. Physically, however, the body is still.

Physical movement and any sleep-walking we do occur during the S phase. Here the brain is washed over by regular waves or pulses of electrical activity.

Pulse, respiration, blood pressure and urine production all fall during the S state, but are higher and more irregular during the D state. Many D periods are accompanied by erections of the penis in the human male, irrespective of dream content. S sleep takes up about 75 per cent of our night and the D stage the remaining 25 per cent.

It was discovered in the late 1950s that our sleep pattern is cyclical. We do not fall into progressively deeper sleep and then wake up again by going through the stages in the reverse order. We go back and forth through stages one to four, four or five times a night; that is, we alternate between S and D sleep in cycles of about one and a half hours. The deeper sleep occurs in the early part of the night. Towards morning we spend more time in the shallower dream state.

The length of this D/S cycle is inversely related to the basal metabolic rate (BMR) of the animal. Small animals like mice have a high BMR and a low cycle time (5 minutes). Elephants have a lower BMR (though only just lower than that of man) and a higher cycle time (100 minutes).

There is also an interesting difference in this D/S pattern with age. A newborn baby will spend only about six hours of its day awake; of its sleep time, ten hours are spent in the dream (D) state and eight hours in sound sleep (S). In the adult, about sixteen and a half hours of the day are spent awake, six hours in sound sleep, and one and a half hours dreaming. You will see that the amount of time spent soundly sleeping has varied little: it is the proportion spent dreaming that has almost disappeared. Although comparatively little time is spent in dream (REM) sleep, its presence in our sleep cycle is nonetheless vital for good health. These two states of sleep are found only in mammals.

Why do we need sleep?

When clinical tests are carried out on young healthy subjects to assess the effects of sleep deprivation, it is difficult to find any significant changes in measured performance. We seem to have the capacity to make a greater mental effort to overcome the physical handicap of drowsiness. The most obvious effect is some deterioration in the power of concentration, and as we get older this effect becomes more marked if we don't get enough sleep. Our body's mental and physical reserves to overcome the problem of sleeplessness are diminished with age. The extreme case of total sleep deprivation in animals causes death.

That we need sleep should scarcely be in question: but there is one theory, however, that suggests we don't – that we sleep mainly out of evolutionary habit. Let's work here on the majority view that sleep is necessary. What do we do with it?

Current thinking suggests that the S stage, deep sleep, is for physical repair to the body. During D stage dreaming, we seem to be re-sorting information, perhaps cleaning the brain's memory store of unwanted material; and generating a sense of well-being. This may be the time when we consolidate learning and balance the emotions if we are disturbed by stress.

How much sleep do we need?

The average sleep requirement for an adult is six to eight hours a night, but there are great variations. Some people need rather longer; many more can manage with much less. The need for longer sleep is not a sign of laziness, nor should short sleepers be regarded as neurotic. Many people function perfectly well in good health on three to four hours' sleep each night. We all have individual sleep needs.

The amount of sleep we need doesn't vary significantly with race, climate, or hours of daylight. Studies on Eskimos or African natives, or subjects in a controlled environment, produce the same general sleep pattern with a similar range of variations.

Many of the great men and women throughout history have been either short or long sleepers. Einstein was a noted long sleeper, Dickens an insomniac. As a generalization, long sleepers tend to be creative, artistic, critical, socially and politically aware, anxious, discontented or moderately neurotic. Short sleepers are more likely to be men and women of action, dynamic, energetic, ambitious, confident, secure and satisfied with life. Whether the personality generates the sleep pattern or vice versa, or whether both arise from some third factor, isn't known.

Sleep patterns seem to be established in infancy, so it's no good trying to force an active child who is quite healthy on six hours' sleep a night, to stay in bed for ten hours. Provided the child is not hyperactive in other ways or obviously ill, the extra time awake and surplus energy can be channelled creatively into other activities.

If you suffer from insomnia, the first rule is not to worry about it. Worry, or stress of any kind, is the most frequent cause of sleeplessness; paradoxically, worry often generates a need for much more sleep, because it saps so much of our energy and we need extra running repairs to our nervous system. So under stress, you may feel you need to sleep more, but are able to sleep less.

If you have problems in sleeping, you should first ask yourself whether you need more sleep. Are you really physically and mentally exhausted, or do you just think that you *ought* to spend more time sleeping because your partner or friends do? The adult sleep pattern doesn't usually become established until maturity in the early 20s, so you can't base your adult sleep needs on what you were used to as a child. Teenagers in particular, while they are growing, usually need a lot more sleep than when they become adults. So if you are happy and healthy, and are not getting overtired on four or five hours' sleep a night, fine – don't worry about it.

The sleep need may decrease by a further hour or two a night as we go from our early 20s to the 70s and 80s, at least partly because we are less active as we grow older, and our BMR decreases.

If you have taken these facts into consideration but still feel you need more sleep, we'll look at a few more practical hints in the next section.

Practical hints on sleeping

The first essential is to relax and not to worry. This is much easier said than achieved. We all have problems to face at various times in our lives, but worrying about them doesn't resolve them or make them disappear.

If you're tired, you are not in the best mental or physical condition to look at problems clearly and objectively. Try to tackle the difficulty when you can do so most effectively, that is, when you're bright, alert and unstressed.

If you are in a relaxed state, even though it may be the middle of the night, make use of the quiet and solitude for some creative thinking. If you're too tired, try to put the issue aside until the morning.

If you cannot put the problem out of your mind and it's preventing you sleeping, think about it constructively to the point where you reach some decision – even if it's only to put it off until you can talk to somebody or get further information. Then *forget it* and concentrate on sleeping. Sleep will put you in better shape to face the obstacle afresh in the morning.

If you're the sort of person who regularly does creative thinking at night, keep a paper and pencil by your bed, jot the ideas down as they come, and then you can forget them. That way, they'll still be there in the morning.

The other point about thinking of problems in bed when you should be sleeping is that you may be facing them on your own. Generally, people find that it helps to talk to someone. It clarifies your own thinking to express your thoughts to someone else, and that person might have experience or just a different point of view which can help you.

If you have no specific worries but relaxation is the problem, yoga or transcendental meditation might show you the way. There are day or evening classes in many major centres now and there you can share your interest with other people.

Try to set aside an hour or so before you go to bed to relax and unwind from the pressures of the day. If you want to relax at home, music or reading may help. The choice of music should be appropriate: something warm and romantic or gently pastoral. If you choose to read, romances or adventure stories are good escapist material; detective or horror stories are more likely to excite than calm you. Books of short stories can also be useful here. The tales come in various lengths and they don't have that 'I couldn't put it down' syndrome you may find with a novel – you can keep reading until you finish a story. Poetry is also good late at night, if you enjoy it. It usually has rhyme and rhythm and this in itself can be relaxing.

Many people find a hot drink at night relaxing, especially one that is milk-based, but tea or coffee late at night should be avoided if possible as they both contain nerve stimulants and diuretics. Some people find an alcoholic drink makes them sleepy, but it's unwise to develop this as a nightly habit.

A heavy meal before bed is not to be recommended, either for the digestion or as an aid to sleeping. Food will be passed onwards through the gut whatever your body position, but as the general direction is downwards from mouth to rectum, standing or sitting is better than lying so that gravity can lend a helping hand to digestion. On the other hand, you don't want to have hunger pangs keeping you awake in the night. A substantial meal not later than six to seven o'clock, or a very light meal at eight is ideal.

Some people find that vigorous exercise just before bedtime makes them so tired that they sleep better. Most of us, however, find this arousing rather than soothing; but you can only try it for yourself and find out. It has to be fairly strenuous exercise, like a jog around the park. Gentle exercise is stimulating to nearly everyone. However, if you tend to be cold in bed, a little exercise for five or ten minutes will help to get the circulation through to the extremities before you lie down.

For light sleepers or those on shift work sleeping during the day, many medical appliance stores and some chemists sell eyeshades to keep out the light, and wax earplugs to shut out the noise.

Temperature in bed at night is more important than in the daytime. When we are awake, we can do things to cool down or warm ourselves up, but when we're asleep, we're on automatic pilot. Make sure you have the right number of bedclothes to keep you at a comfortable temperature. Use a hot water bottle or electric blanket if you have difficulty in staying warm. Despite the current controversy over infra-red cookers, there has never been the slightest suggestion that the infra-red radiation from electric blankets is in any way harmful, and they've been around a lot longer. Don't forget that foam pillows and foam or wool mattresses will keep you a lot warmer than feather pillows or spring mattresses.

Bed size is another important and sometimes vexed question. Some people are more secure in small beds, while others like room to thrash around in. Some are so restless they disturb their night-time partners, while others move scarcely at all during the night. You have to weigh up possible advantages of not disturbing or being disturbed by your mate against possible lack of emotional closeness when you opt for single or double beds.

You also want a bed that is firm enough to give support to your skeleton when all the muscles are relaxed. Foam mattresses may seem very comfortable in the furniture showroom, as you sink luxuriously into them and disappear from sight. Sleeping on them every night, however, is likely to give you aches and pains in places you didn't even know you had muscles. Going to the other extreme, an orthopedic bed which may provide nocturnal bliss for some will shut off the blood supply for others, producing the familiar tingling of 'pins and needles' as those limbs join in the body circulation once more. There's no rule about this: you have to find out by trial and error just what suits you. But this, or any other one of the factors mentioned above, can make the difference between a calm, refreshed start to each new day and a dread of watching the sun creep up yet again above the yardarm.

Let's deal briefly with the topic of sleeping pills. These may be prescribed by your family doctor or obtained as the herbal variety from health supplies stores. Although the latter are less powerful, they are all drugs and can produce dependence if used for long periods.

If you need to take sleeping pills to see you through an emotional crisis, you should do so for no more than three or four weeks, and then come off them gradually. If they are in tablet form, take one-half then one-quarter of a tablet each night until you can give them up entirely. If they are capsules, take one every other night, then every third night, and so on, to wean yourself off them. After three or four weeks' continuous use, sleeping pills appear to have little effect on the sleep centre of the brain. After that, most of their soporific effect is psychosomatic or autosuggestive – you just think you need them and that they're still doing you some good. If you take them for a really long time, you may never be able to give them up. Vitamin B may be an effective long-term alternative.

Part 3

THE BODY IN DISEASE

17
DRUGS

With only a quick glance at the title of this chapter, some readers might hurry on, thinking that it is not relevant as far as they are concerned. Yet many people who wouldn't think of taking so much as an aspirin still get regular daily doses of drugs.

A drug may be thought of as a compound foreign to the body, which is not part of a natural biochemical nutrient system but which has a detectable physiological effect that may be made use of in medicine. In the widest sense of the term, all those substances which have no medicinal use but to which the other parts of the definition still apply should be included.

The majority of people, unless they abstain for some religious or health reason, take non-medicinal stimulating drugs regularly and eagerly every day in order to see them through from dawn to dusk: tea, coffee, cocoa, cola drinks, tobacco and alcohol all fall into this category.

One prominent religious group which shuns all such artificial stimulants is the Mormons. The Church of Jesus Christ of Latter Day Saints, founded in the US in 1830, is concentrated in the state of Utah in America. Health statistics for this state show a smaller-than-average incidence of heart disease, strokes, cancer of the gut or lung, and sclerosis of the liver. With what is now known about the physiologically damaging effects of cigarettes and stimulating drinks, the correlation of health with abstinence is not unexpected.

Let's now take a look at each of these groups of drugs in turn.

TEA, COFFEE, COCOA AND COLA

We'll consider these drinks together since pharmacologically they have much in common. Teas are in fact infusions of the leaves of plants; coffees come from the plant roots or seeds (beans).

History

Tea originated in the Orient, probably in China, and has been widely used there for at least 2,000 years. Locally it is known as *t'e* or *ch'a*, which gives the colloquial word for the drink. It was introduced first into continental Europe and then into England by Dutch explorers during the latter half of the seventeenth century. There is no reference to tea in the Bible, and none in Shakespeare or other literary works in English before this time.

The drinking of coffee began in Arabia, perhaps as recently as 500 years ago, and then spread to England and the rest of Europe also in the seventeenth century. The first English coffee houses opened in the 1650s in Oxford and London, and tea was introduced there soon after, together with cocoa from Central and South America. Cocoa beans were used by the Mayas and Aztecs as a source of food and drink, as well as serving as a medium of exchange in trading. Solid chocolate also made its first appearance in London, again in the seventeenth century, but eating chocolate as a sweet didn't come into vogue until the nineteenth century.

The coca plant was used as a stimulant by the Incas and is derived from the same geographical region as cocoa. It was an ingredient in Coca-Cola until its use was banned in 1904. The beans from which cola drinks are prepared came originally from Africa, but they are now grown extensively throughout the Tropics, especially in South America.

Active ingredients and their properties

The tea plant is an evergreen, known botanically as *Camellia sp.* (formerly *Thea sp.*) and it is grown mainly in Asia where it is favoured by the hot, humid climate.

In preparing black tea, the leaves are dried and fermented before packing, but leaves for green tea are steamed to prevent fermentation. The leaves of the third type of tea, oolong tea, are semi-fermented. The characteristic flavour is due to chemicals called *polyphenols* or *tannins*, the nature and quantity of which are highly dependent on this fermentation process.

Coffee beans are the roasted seeds of various species of the evergreen Coffea trees, now grown mainly in Africa and South America. The roasting process changes the sugars into *caramel* (which is the common name for burnt sugar), the starch into smaller carbohydrate units called *dextrins*, and reduces appreciably the *caffeine* content of the beans. It is these chemical changes that contribute to the overall flavour and aroma of the ultimate coffee brew.

Cocoa is prepared from the seeds of *Theobroma cacao* and is the distinctive ingredient in chocolate. The seeds are fermented and roasted before drying and commercial packaging.

Although cocoa contains a little caffeine, the main active ingredient is *theobromine*. Tea and coffee both contain a significant amount (100 to 150 mg per cup) of caffeine and tea has *theophylline* in addition. All these compounds belong to the same chemical family (*xanthine alkaloids*), and all are nerve stimulants (*analeptics*) – caffeine the greatest, theobromine the least. They are all also heart stimulants and diuretics, that is, they increase the desire to empty the bladder; in this respect, theophylline is the most powerful and caffeine the weakest. Caffeine is completely absorbed in the small intestine, and most of it is converted into urea and carbon dioxide.

On the positive side, tea is rich in minerals (potassium, manganese and fluoride) and vitamins (A, B, E and K), but there are no such nutrients in coffee. A process was devised in Germany at the turn of the century for removing most of the caffeine from coffee by treating it with chlorinated organic solvents. In view of the extreme toxicity of these compounds, however, it is a moot point which is likely to do us more harm – all the original caffeine or traces of solvent residue which may remain after processing.

Cola drinks contain about 20 to 35 mg of caffeine in a 250 ml bottle, about one-fifth the content of a cup of tea or coffee. The beans come from the Cola tree, *Sterculia acuminata*, a close relation botanically of the cocoa tree, *Theobroma*, and one which looks somewhat like a horse chestnut.

The active ingredient of the coca plant (*Erythroxylum coca*) is *cocaine* (a *tropane alkaloid*), which is obtained from the leaves. Cocaine is a stimulant of the central nervous system, producing restlessness and euphoria. It was the drug used by Sherlock Holmes to sharpen his mind for his most difficult cases. It is also a nasal and bronchial decongestant, and a surface and local anaesthetic. The coca leaf is still widely used as a stimulant in Chile, India and Sri Lanka; the leaves are generally dried and chewed.

Ill effects

We have seen that tea, coffee, cocoa and cola all contain stimulating drugs. Excessive tea or coffee drinking causes nervous irritability, sleeplessness, gastritis and palpitations of the heart. The question is: what is excessive? Some people experience these effects with only one or two cups; others can take ten cups or more a day without any problem. You have to assess your own limits, but if you know what to look for you can adjust your intake accordingly.

There has recently been some evidence that excessive coffee drinking may also be associated with stomach cancer and an increased incidence of heart disease, but causative factors have not yet been established. There is no evidence at present that tea provokes similar symptoms.

Alternatives

For those who wish to avoid any potential ill effects of tea or coffee, there are many alternative infusions for the preparation of hot drinks.

Teas are commonly prepared from sumac (*Rhus sp.*), wintergreen (*Gaultheria procumbens*), caraway (*Carum carvi*), chamomile *(Matricaria chamomilla*), rosemary (*Rosmarinus officinalis*) or lime (*Tilia cordata*), to mention but a few.

Coffees from the seeds of hawthorn (*Crataegus oxycantha*) or asparagus (*Asparagus officinalis*), or from the roots of dandelions (*Taraxacum officinalis*) are available from many health supplies stores.

Carob (*Jacaranda procera*) is a common substitute for cocoa and chocolate.

ALCOHOL

The drinking of fermented liquors prepared from starch or sugar goes back thousands of years to the earliest civilizations, though it wasn't until about 1500 BC that yeast was added to generate fermentation instead of leaving the process to the chance invasion of airborne spores. Ever since its discovery, alcohol has been used for social, religious and medicinal purposes.

Alcohol is probably the oldest of the drugs that we come across in everyday life. As all grains and potatoes contain starch and all fruits varying amounts of starch and sugar, there are many readily available sources of fermentation material. Starch cannot be fermented directly but must first be converted to the single-unit sugars. These are changed by enzymes in yeast to alcohols with the liberation of carbon dioxide. A mixture of alcohols is then produced, the composition of which depends on the nature of the fermentation material, but the main one is called *ethanol*.

In the case of cereals, the alcoholic product is called beer. Grapes and other plants produce varieties of wine. Wine that is changed biochemically by the action of a mould known as flor is denoted as sherry, a name derived from Jerez in Spain where the process originated. A blend of mature wines which originated in Oporto, Portugal, is called port. Most wines contain 10 to 12 per cent alcohol, but sherry and port may have up to 20 per cent, having been fortified with pure alcohol. Beers, on the other hand, have less than 10 per cent alcohol; lager, a light beer, usually has less than 5 per cent.

The fermentation process alone can never produce a brew with more than about 15 per cent alcohol because at higher concentrations the alcohol kills the activity of the yeast. If alcohol concentrations in the 20 to 70 per cent range are required, the fermented liquor must be distilled. This gives rise to other ranges of alcoholic beverages: spirits and liqueurs.

The distinction between these two groups should be clear-cut, but both terms are applied to some drinks. The fortification by distillation produces a *spirit*. A *liqueur* is a spirit which has been sweetened with up to 50 per cent sugar and flavoured and perfumed by herbs, spices or fruits. The various drinks differ in their starting material and flavouring.

Mead is derived from honey, rum from molasses. Gin is flavoured in the distillation process by juniper berries; the French name for these is *genièvre* and this has become shortened and anglicized to 'gin'. Brandy begins with fruit, usually grapes, for fermentation, though some European varieties are derived from other fruits.

There are many other regional varieties of spirit. Scotch whisky and Irish whiskey start from barley and corn, the Scotch being dried with peat, which gives it its distinctive earthy flavour. Russian vodka is prepared from fermented potatoes, Mexican tequila starts from cactus, and Japanese saki is made from rice.

There are thus many different varieties of alcoholic drink containing not only a mixture of alcohols but also various flavourings. Once in the body, alcohol is rapidly absorbed by the stomach and intestine and passed into the blood stream. Most of the alcohol is oxidized by enzymes in the liver, ultimately forming acetic acid, or carbon dioxide and water with the liberation of energy (about 7 kcal/g alcohol).

Ill effects

Physiologically, alcohol is a depressant: the apparent excitant effect experienced on drinking alcohol is due to depression of inhibitory systems in the higher centres of the brain. It has been used medicinally for centuries as a mild sedative and anaesthetic.

One of the effects that alcohol has on the body is to cause a relaxation of the muscle walls of our blood vessels, allowing them to widen (*vasodilation*). This results in the characteristic glow when we take an alcoholic drink; it improves the peripheral circulation and warms us when we come in from the cold. However, alcohol shouldn't be used for warming when going out into the cold from a warm environment because the widened blood vessels and capillaries near the surface of the skin will expose warm blood to cold temperatures. The reason we go pale when we are cold is because the capillaries contract to keep the blood deeper inside our warm bodies.

The nausea which is experienced with excessive drinking is due to irritation of the lining of the stomach (*gastritis*). The headache of a hangover arises from a combination of hypersensitivity to the additives and alcohol congeners, and the toxicity of the alcohol itself. Weight gain as a result of drinking arises from the unchanged carbohydrates ingested with the alcohol and from the use of the alcohol as fuel instead of the body's reserve fat.

An alcohol concentration of as little as 50 mg/100 ml blood is enough to produce some deterioration in performance in most people, unless they are habitual drinkers. At a concentration of 150 mg/100 ml your mood can best be described as 'merry'. At 250 mg/100 ml speech is slurred, vision is blurred and co-ordination is poor. At 350 mg/100 ml you will be dead drunk, and at 450 mg/100 ml probably dead. In Europe and the US there are restrictions on blood alcohol levels for driving, which vary from zero in some countries to 80 mg/100 ml in the UK.

Excessive intake of alcohol produces a deficiency of vitamins B1 and C (leading to degeneration of the nerves and trembling, a condition described as delirium tremens – DTs); increased susceptibility to infection because of interference with the body's capacity to make white blood cells; increased deposition of lipids in the liver (producing a fatty liver and ultimately *cirrhosis*); indigestion and inadequate food absorption both from gastric irritation and because the liver cannot make bile acids effectively; and thence general damage indirectly to all systems of the body.

Alcohol is a poison and it can easily become addictive – not so much physiologically as for its effects on mood and behaviour. If it is taken in small doses, the healthy body can cope without difficulty, but the more you drink, the more you tax the system. If you are smoking or taking drugs as well it is the cumulative effect of all these toxins that you have to consider. Under no circumstances should you ever take alcohol with barbiturates or antihistamines, or other depressants of the central nervous system – the combined effect can be fatal. For healthy living, it is a drug we should ingest very sparingly.

TOBACCO

Perhaps the most lethal of all the drugs we take on a regular basis are those we derive from tobacco, whether chewed, sniffed or smoked. The case against coffee is still largely circumstantial; and although some of the ingredients in tea may be detrimental to our health, there are others which are undoubtedly beneficial; but with smoking, unfortunately, the news is all bad.

Smoking damages the body in a number of ways. In the depths of the lungs there are tiny sacs (*alveoli*) which fill with air. Oxygen in the air is vital for the life of every cell in the body; without oxygen cells die. The tar in tobacco smoke clogs up these air sacs so that they can no longer function. All cells in the body are thus affected by the decrease in oxygen supply: vitality is diminished and health deteriorates.

Tar from burnt tobacco, like the tar from burnt wood or coal, contains a number of substances that promote cancer (*carcinogens*).

Heavy smokers are therefore liable to cancer of those organs which come into contact with the tobacco smoke – the mouth, throat and lungs.

When any organic substance is burned, the products of burning are oxides of carbon and water. If there is enough oxygen about carbon dioxide is formed, but if there isn't enough oxygen then carbon monoxide is the result. This is one of the deadliest ingredients in car exhaust fumes. It is also a major constituent of tobacco smoke.

Oxygen in the lungs is carried to cells in other parts of the body by the blood. The carrier is the substance that gives red blood cells their colour (*haemoglobin*). Oxygen combines chemically with this carrier in the lungs and is plucked off again as needed by the tissues. Carbon monoxide, however, combines with the carrier in a way that the body cannot reverse. The carrier is effectively taken out of circulation so that it cannot go back and fetch more oxygen. So a daily diet of carbon monoxide, whether from tobacco smoke or car exhaust, further diminishes the oxygen supply to the cells. As a result, the heart works harder to try to correct the oxygen deficiency, and in this way smoking produces a strain on the heart.

Finally, there is nicotine. Even one filter cigarette may contain 20 to 30 mg of nicotine, some 10 per cent of which is absorbed by inhalation of the smoke. It is only slowly degraded by the body and stimulates the nervous system. By so doing, it produces a temporary feeling of well-being. Once this has worn off, the nervous system calls for another dose – the craving for tobacco, which leads ultimately to addiction, has begun. This is why it's so difficult to give up smoking once you have started. Nicotine is, in fact, more addictive than either alcohol or barbiturates, so smokers should not chastise themselves too much when they find it so hard to give up the habit: it isn't purely psychological.

Giving up smoking

The link between smoking and ill health – cancer, heart disease, bronchitis and emphysema – is now so well established that it is no longer statistical conjecture. Long before its effects are terminal, smoking saps our strength. Anything that we can do to cut down on smoking has got to be a plus if we are serious about our health.

Although a lot of people may want to give up, they find that they can't. One treatment that might be of help is a course of hypnosis. Many people have been cured by this method, although it doesn't work for everyone.

In the short term, there is also a special chewing gum available which contains *lobeline* (a nicotine-related alkaloid from *Lobelia inflata*). This is intended to break you gently out of the habit. If you chew this stuff for long enough, however, it can become as addictive as the cigarettes, but at least it is nothing like as harmful as the tobacco smoke. Nor do you pollute the atmosphere for everyone around you.

There is no doubt that if you spend a significant amount of time in a smoke-filled atmosphere, even though you don't smoke yourself, you will inhale toxins just as you would by smoking. Of course, you won't get as large a dose, but even short exposure may still produce the starchy, watery eyes and sore throat which indicate the smoke toxins are having their effect (passive smoking).

The question of banning smoking in public places is currently a matter of debate. There are those who see this as another encroachment on civil liberties of the individual, but there are undoubtedly many people who find tobacco smoke highly irritating. In a free society each of us has a right to do as he pleases, provided that what we do is not to the detriment of other people. That is not tolerated even in primitive societies. Just as smokers feel they have a right to smoke if they wish, so non-smokers have an equal right to breathe smoke-free air. If aversion to tobacco smoke were merely a personal whim, then the question of unwanted exposure would not be so critical. But evidence of the damage that inhaling even other people's smoke can do is now irrefutable. Perhaps the time has come for all public places to have smoking and non-smoking areas, as there now are in buses, trains and planes. Then everyone can surround themselves with whatever environment they choose.

The most pressing need is for education of the young so that they don't start smoking in the first place. It is so much easier not to start than to try to stop. Pointing out the health hazards in a general way doesn't appear to be effective: children must be well aware of these by now. A more personal appeal seems to have more impact, but with the financial support of sports and the arts increasingly assumed by cigarette manufacturers, and with ever greater revenues from tobacco duty, it is not in a government's interest in the short term to inhibit smoking amongst any sector of the population. Only if ultimate savings in health care costs are taken into account is there any hope of making the argument for anti-smoking education more persuasive to an Exchequer. Participation in schemes of preventive medicine is not likely to be attractive otherwise. Politicians, unfortunately, seem to be more concerned with votes and expediency than with ethics, altruism or long-term benefits.

PHARMACEUTICAL DRUGS

Finally, we should take a look at those drugs which are taken for a specific ailment, concentrating on those that are available at a chemist without prescription.

Analgesics for pain

Pain is the body's way of telling us something is wrong. The ideal response to pain, therefore, should always be to try to identify and eliminate the source.

Stomach pain and back pain (see also Chapter 12) will be dealt with separately. Let's concentrate here on headaches, which are the main reason for taking painkillers, and consider some of the factors that may be responsible for them.

Stress is one of the main causes of headaches. Examine your life style for obvious sources: a pressured job; noisy or demanding children; tension in relationships with spouse, relatives, or neighbours; emotional, sexual or mental frustration. Some of these problems may be easy to resolve, others more difficult, but in any event a continual supply of painkillers is not a satisfactory answer. The pain may not even be adequately suppressed and the demand for drugs often increases with use. Eliminating the source of tension, or at least reducing it to a tolerable level, is the only long-term solution.

If you are a woman, headaches are often a part of pre-menstrual tension, usually experienced in the latter half of the cycle (days 14 to 28 or thereabouts). Some people have found relief from all symptoms with daily doses of from 40 to 80 mg of vitamin B6 (pyridoxine). Relaxation therapy, such as you get in yoga or meditation classes, may help this or any other tension situation. If you have abdominal cramps associated with a period, general massage of the abdomen for five to ten minutes night and morning over the tender region, pressing firmly but gently on the uterus or ovaries, will often ease the pain.

If you are male or are not under any great stress, you need to look for other possible sources of headache: excessive drinking of alcohol or coffee, working in a room with poor lighting or ventilation, insufficient exercise (and therefore too little oxygen in the system), constipation, or problems with eyesight should be considered.

Monosodium glutamate, a food additive widely used to enhance flavour and particularly abundant in some Oriental dishes and tinned soups, is renowned for producing headache as well as nausea and stomach cramps in susceptible individuals.

If headaches are only occasional, one of several types of painkiller or *analgesic* can be used. Aspirin *(acetylsalicylic acid)* is one of the longest-serving. In excess it may produce some bleeding from the wall of the gut, but this seems to be minimized by the use of the soluble varieties. Aspirin is widely used for rheumatic and arthritic pain since it has an anti-inflammatory effect through its reaction with prostaglandins, in addition to its analgesic properties.

A combination of aspirin with codeine is even more effective in

104

clearing pain, and this is also available in soluble form.

Paracetamol is one of the newer analgesics. It is recommended particularly for those who suffer from peptic ulcers when aspirin cannot be used, but it is also not without side effects since it taxes the liver.

Antacids for indigestion

Prevention is always better than cure and if you can track down your indigestion to a particular food or type of food so much the better. You will then know what to avoid (or expect!) in future. Fruit juice, alcohol, coffee, shellfish, dishes with a high spice or fat content (especially animal fats like suet), or Oriental food containing monosodium glutamate should always be regarded as suspects.

If the deed is done, however, and you and your rebellious stomach have to live together for the next few hours, there are many mild and simple home remedies.

Bicarbonate of soda (*sodium bicarbonate*) is rapid-acting, but its effect is short-lived; frequent use may produce alkalosis with headache and drowsiness, and it builds up the sodium content of the body, which is not considered desirable.

You should, if possible, avoid proprietary antacids which contain sodium: the sodium-free brands are usually mixtures of the carbonates of calcium and magnesium. A spearmint or peppermint flavouring also has a carminative effect (see page 138). Similarly, in view of what has been said about the gastric irritation produced by aspirin, you should be careful to avoid any stomach powders which contain this drug.

Milk of magnesia (a suspension of *magnesium oxide* and *hydroxide*) is effective – slower to work but longer-lasting than bicarbonate of soda. The main disadvantage is that it tends to cause diarrhoea. Calcium carbonate used as an antacid may have the reverse effect and produce constipation. Calcium and magnesium compounds used together are ideal.

Bismuth salts are used in some antacids on the principle that they will line and protect the inflamed gut wall. It is not established, however, that this effect does indeed occur to an extent sufficient to reduce indigestion.

Antacids are useful for combating indigestion only if it arises because of excess acid in the gut – and this is by no means always the case. This is why it is always important to identify the cause of your indigestion. If it arises from something like alcohol or fatty food, an antacid will be almost completely ineffective.

Antibiotics and antiseptics for infection

The chemical compounds known as *phenols* are widely used as mild antiseptics. They were first employed by Lister a century ago and various members of the phenol family are applied externally or taken internally. Note, however, that many of these compounds are highly toxic and corrosive, and they should *never* be used internally unless directed. Some throat pastilles contain a non-toxic phenol.

Minor cuts and abrasions can also be safely treated with *zinc oxide* ointment; zinc oxide powder or ointment will help to prevent nappy rash, or the development of odour or the fungal infection known as athlete's foot in perspiring feet. Bites and stings often respond to calamine (*zinc carbonate*), usually applied as a lotion.

In the case of serious systemic infection it may be necessary to use antibiotics to kill the invading bacteria. *Penicillins, cephalosporins* and *tetracyclines* are all prescribed for this purpose. These chemicals, which are themselves produced by moulds and bacteria, have no effect on viruses such as those which cause colds, influenza, or common childhood ailments like measles, mumps or chickenpox. They act against secondary bacteria which generate the nasal and bronchial congestion associated with many viral diseases.

When they are utilized, antibiotics must be taken three or four times a day for four to six days to build up a sufficiently high blood concentration to kill the bacteria. They do tend to kill the friendly little germs we have in our gut at the same time, so constipation, diarrhoea, indigestion and irritability are common side effects of their use. Occasionally, by killing our own natural bacteria, they allow hostile fungi to generate, with the development of superinfection.

Because antibiotics are so widely administered to animals, not only to cure their infections but also to promote growth, we ingest significant amounts by consuming animal produce, and this has developed resistance or promoted allergic or hypersensitivity reactions in many individuals.

Tetracyclines tend to form complexes (*chelates*) with metal ions such as magnesium, calcium or iron. This reaction (known as *chelation*) inactivates the drugs in the body, so you should avoid milk, antacids or iron tablets within at least two or three hours (and preferably longer) of taking tetracycline medication.

As an alternative to antibiotics like terramycin or chloromycin, when they are prescribed for conjunctivitis (inflammation of the eyelid), the 'old-fashioned' remedy of *boracic* or *boric acid* solution might prove effective. Provided it is only used externally and never on open wounds, it is a mild antiseptic, cheap and soothing, and it does not deteriorate with age.

Antihistamines for rhinitis and sympathomimetics for asthma

An *antihistamine* is a drug that blocks the site of action of histamine, which is released by the intrusion of an *allergen* into our system.

Most antihistamines are available only on prescription from a medical practitioner. There are some brands, however, which can be bought without prescription and which are widely used, even for children, as a remedy for hay fever.

The main disadvantage of many antihistamines is that they cause drowsiness and therefore should never be taken by people who operate machinery or need to drive. Also, they should *never* be taken within four hours of an alcoholic drink, or within twelve hours of an alcoholic spree, as the resulting depression of the central nervous sytem may prove fatal. Although originally intended for the relief of allergic reactions, some antihistamines are now commonly prescribed as sedatives or hypnotics because of their soporific effect.

Antihistamines taken for hay fever may also partially alleviate asthma, but the effect is usually slight. Asthmatics will generally need *sympathomimetics* for their condition. These are drugs which mimic the physiological effects of the stimulation of our *sympathetic nervous system* and the release of *adrenaline*. Common medications of this type are adrenaline itself, injected or inhaled; *ephedrine*, swallowed as tablets; or *isoprenaline*, inhaled or dissolved under the tongue.

Inhalants are popular with asthmatics as they reach the seat of the problem in the lungs directly. There are many single compounds in inert aerosol propellants available as pocket inhalers. Users may encounter problems with some of these, however: with some types of asthma attack, the inhalant will make breathing more difficult momentarily before it brings relief; inhalants may generate dependence with the need for further doses at four- to six-hourly intervals; and they commonly produce palpitations and other symptoms of the anxiety state – sweating, fear, fainting and trembling. It is the now-familiar story of finding what suits you best.

Steroid preparations are used as long-term treatments for asthma and hay fever, but doctors prescribe oral steroids only reluctantly because of their side effects, although they are an extremely effective form of medication.

For rhinitis and allergic asthma, the best remedy is to track down the cause, although this may be far from easy, and eliminating the cause from your environment may prove even more difficult (see Chapter 18).

Soporifics for insomnia

The first synthetic hypnotics were the barbiturates which appeared in the 1890s. A new chemical family of sedatives and soporifics (*benzodiaze-*

pines) was discovered and first used in the 1970s, and two members of this group soon became the most-often prescribed of all drugs. Extracts of passion flower (*Passiflora incarnata*), valerian (*Valeriana officinalis*) and black nightshade (*Solanum americanum*) have long been among the more popular herbal remedies for insomnia.

Remedies for insomnia have been discussed in Chapter 16. If all else fails and you decide to resort to drugs, try to limit their daily use to three or four weeks only. After that, wean yourself off them by taking one capsule every two or three nights, or one-half then one-quarter tablet only, until you can do without them. Most barbiturates and tranquillizers are habit-forming, so they should be taken only to see you through some short-term crisis.

There are many herbal remedies for insomnia, but remember that these are still drugs. They are no different from pharmaceutical preparations in principle except that they are much weaker. The most beneficial and potent ingredient in such herbal tablets is likely to be vitamin B. This vitamin B is in fact a mixture of all the different vitamins known to be beneficial to the nervous system: thiamin (B1), niacin (B3), pantothenate (B5) and pyridoxine (B6). A combination of this vitamin (100 to 200 mg daily), exercise, fresh air and mental relaxation with an adequate diet should enable you to get all the sleep you need, even if it is only four or five hours a night.

Decongestants for catarrh

Herbal mixtures of plant extracts are as effective as most other external treatments for catarrh, and menthol preparations are also popular. Medication for the internal treatment of catarrh often has an antihistamine effect in addition to its decongestant action.

Diuretics for oedema

If there is a build-up of fluid in the body – a condition known as *oedema* – a person may be prescribed diuretics to get the kidneys working more vigorously. Sluggish kidneys are often accompanied by headaches, lethargy, nausea and backache, located just below the ribs and above the hip bone.

Amongst the home remedies is theophylline in tea and, to a lesser degree, the caffeine in tea and coffee; these are both simple and effective. Women may find these useful in countering the fluid build-up which frequently occurs as part of the menstrual cycle. For those who want to avoid the arousal effects of tea or coffee, some of their substitutes, like extract of dandelion roots, are pleasant, safe, non-stimulating and diuretic. Some people find a high-protein diet alone is effective.

As mentioned in Chapter 27, diuresis is always accompanied by loss of soluble mineral salts in the urine. Those on pharmacological diuretic preparations would be well advised to take a tablet mineral supplement.

As oedema may be a symptom of some fundamental disorder, if it does not respond to simple home remedies within a few weeks you should always consult your physician.

Laxatives for constipation

Treatment of constipation with laxatives should be short-term only. Having accepted this, the herbal preparations of cascara or senna can be recommended. Alternatively, magnesium salts, such as may be found in Epsom salts (*magnesium sulphate*) or milk of magnesia (a suspension of magnesium oxide and hydroxide), have a mild laxative effect.

In the long term, increasing intake of dietary fibre and exercising the abdominal muscles are the only satisfactory solutions to constipation. Continual use of laxatives may lead to loss of fluids and mineral salts from the body and produce inflammation of the bowel. The aim should be to have at least one, and not more than three, bowel actions each day without straining.

18
ALLERGY

Introduction

Allergy proper is considered to be a reaction of the body's immune system to a foreign protein, called an *allergen* or *antigen*, which is ingested by inhalation, by injection, or through food.

We've seen in Chapter 5 how some people react against the lactose in milk or the fructose in fruit. There are also people who are allergic to one of the various proteins in milk: *lactalbumin, lactoglobulin, casein* or *bovine serum albumin* (BSA). Allergy to the wheat protein, *gluten*, is well recognized as the cause of *coeliac disease*. Some people are allergic to drugs like penicillin. But the most common sources of allergens are pollen, mould spores, animal fur or feathers, and house dust or dander (skin particles of animals and humans that constitute a significant portion of what we call 'house dust'). The mite that inhabits house dust is also a frequent cause of irritation. For all of these, inhalation is the usual path of entry into the body.

In addition to this type of allergic reaction, there are other adverse reactions which some people experience to a wide variety of substances, often synthetic non-protein products of the twentieth century, such as plastics, solvents and food additives. Non-protein natural products, including many found in otherwise nutritious foods, may also engender such a reaction in some individuals. In the current terminology this reaction is usually called *idiosyncrasy*, *hypersensitivity*, *intolerance* or *susceptibility* rather than allergy, though many people use the term 'allergy' to refer to any such adverse reaction whether it involves proteins or not.

ALLERGY AND ANAPHYLAXIS

Let's deal first with 'classical' allergy, a term which originated with Clemens von Pirquet in 1906. As he defined the term, it applied to adverse reactions which were *acquired* by previous exposure to the allergen. The belief nowadays is that many people are born with this problem and it is assumed that in these cases the genetic susceptibility is inherited by exposure of the foetus to the allergen while still in the womb.

There are three distinct types of allergic reaction which have been recognized:

1 Delayed reaction allergies: there may be no reaction to the initial exposure, which merely sensitizes the system. The allergic reaction comes with any subsequent exposure. Responses to poison oak, poison ivy and to insect stings are examples of this type of allergy.

2 Atopic allergies: these are apparently inherited and they produce inflammation in the tissues (*epithelial tissues*) which line various surfaces of the body when these are exposed to the allergens. The result may be constriction of the air passages (*bronchioles*) leading to the lungs, producing *asthma*; irritation of the nasal linings (*rhinitis*), resulting in copious nasal discharge (*rhinorrhoea*) and sneezing to produce the condition called *hay fever* (though the allergen is usually not hay); and itching (*pruritis*) of the skin with lesions (*eczema*) or swellings to produce *hives* (*urticaria*).

Typically, these allergens are identified by skin tests: pricking the surface of the skin with a solution of the suspected allergen. If we are allergic to it, this will produce a raised weal, the size of the swelling being taken as a measure of the degree of allergy to that substance. The tests are unreliable, however, since the reaction that an allergen produces in the skin may be quite different from that which is produced if it is inhaled into the nose and lungs or ingested into the stomach.

The usual treatment for these conditions is to try to desensitize patients by injecting them with successively larger doses of the allergen, the theory being that the immune system is increasingly stimulated to respond to the maximum natural dose to which the individual may then be exposed in the environment. As the problem arises in the first place because of a defective immune system, the desensitization procedure often overloads the immune system intolerably, producing no immunity and acute reaction to the antigen on subsequent exposure. The allergic symptoms are usually controlled during the course of treatment only by the use of strong drugs. When these are withdrawn, the symptoms frequently reappear. Desensitization is therefore only moderately successful.

Most of the drugs which are used to treat one form of allergic response are usually ineffective in combating another. Steroid drugs are highly effective in treating several allergies simultaneously, but their long-term use gives rise to complications.

3 Precipitin allergies: in this group of allergic reactions the allergen stimulates the immune system enough to produce some antibodies, which then combine with the particular antigen to form a precipitate – the complex is no longer soluble in body fluids. As such reactions may occur within the tissues, these are potentially the most dangerous of allergic responses.

Anaphylactic shock is one such reaction and this produces low blood pressure, disturbance of the heart rhythm, and oedema. The reaction some people have to penicillin is of this type, and without immediate treatment it is frequently fatal. Reaction to foreign blood serum after transfusion is another precipitin reaction, though this usually develops more slowly than anaphylaxis, and is therefore more easily remedied.

ENVIRONMENTAL SUSCEPTIBILITY

Now we move into a much more controversial area, but one which is slowly gaining acceptance by orthodox medical practitioners. This is the field of *clinical ecology*, also known as *environmental medicine*. Ecology is the study of plants and animals in their natural environment; clinical ecology is the study of humans in their environment, particularly with regard to the ways in which they react against it.

The problems

As we have seen in Chapter 5, there are millions of people throughout the world who have an intolerance to substances as simple and natural as lactose and fructose: these are now medically recognized conditions. Yet so many orthodox medical practitioners, and particularly allergy specialists, still refuse to accept that there may be many millions more people who cannot tolerate other natural foodstuffs or the totally foreign and frequently toxic substances to which they are exposed in the environment. This environmental susceptibility or hypersensitivity is usually dismissed as psychosomatic or emotional in origin, which may indeed account for some cases, but its apparently widespread occurrence in otherwise normal and well-adjusted individuals implies that this is unlikely to be the causative factor in all cases. In recent years, accepted scientific methods of investigation, including double-blind trials in which neither the patient nor the experimenter has known the nature of the substances being administered, have ruled out the psychosomatic possibility as a cause with many of the patients who have been successfully treated.

One of the reasons why these ideas have not been readily accepted is the issue of terminology. Allergy has been thought of only as a response of the immune system to foreign proteins. The fact that so many non-proteins can produce demonstrable adverse effects was regarded as evidence that it wasn't 'allergy', though the antigen-immune system reaction was never part of von Pirquet's concept of allergy.

Another problem is that the range of symptoms produced is much wider than those associated with classical allergy – often so many in one individual as to lead to the diagnosis of nervous or emotional disorder.

Medical science is traditionally very conservative. New ideas, especially ones as revolutionary as these – that simple substances in food or common toxins in the environment could cause such a wide range of illnesses – are bound to meet with considerable opposition.

Perhaps one of the most powerful and most unfortunate arguments against acceptance of the food and environmental allergy concept is the financial one. If such allergy is ultimately proven to be the cause of more than 50 per cent of the illnesses currently being treated by drugs (and this is the sort of proportion that many clinical ecologists *are* treating successfully), then the loss of revenue to the pharmaceutical companies would be enormous. These companies sponsor many of the medical journals which should be publishing the results of these researches, but don't. Pharmaceutical companies also fund a great deal of medical research and contribute towards the salaries of researchers, so it is certainly not in their interests to have this philosophy promoted widely. This is not cynicism: it is plain, economic fact. Every drug company would lose profits; some would face financial ruin if their products were no longer used because people were being cured simply, cheaply, and without side effects, merely by abstaining from one or more foods or by eliminating a toxin from their environment. The battle has a long way to go yet.

The effects

Researchers in this field maintain that *any person* can become sensitized to foreign substances, including foodstuffs, if they are ingested in large enough quantities at frequent intervals, and that *any substance* may produce adverse reactions in otherwise healthy people if they are susceptible. The precise amount of compound needed to provoke response will vary greatly from person to person and, more frustratingly, will vary from one time to another even in the same individual, depending on other factors.

The most common effects of environmental allergy are nervous disorders such as headache, irritability, fatigue, palpitations, depression or insomnia, and ultimately convulsions; and digestive troubles such as indigestion, heartburn, flatulence, nausea, diarrhoea or constipation, or a combination of symptoms known as irritable bowel syndrome. Sudden and otherwise inexplicable changes of mood are often associated with this type of allergy. Some cases of arthritis, multiple sclerosis, and other joint and muscle disorders have been successfully treated by food or pollutant elimination from the patient's environment. Exposure to food or environmental allergens may also give rise to the classical allergic responses of asthma, hay fever, eczema and hives.

These symptoms may arise in any of three ways:

1   They may be caused by the initial exposure to the allergen.
2   They may be the result of a build-up effect if intake is maintained.
3   They may arise as withdrawal symptoms if the exposure is stopped after prolonged intake.

In testing for the cause of adverse reactions, a person is withdrawn from exposure for three or four days and then each potential problem substance is introduced one at a time to see if an adverse reaction develops.

In the case of food allergy, the foods may produce a stimulating effect or craving, resulting in a compulsion to eat that which is doing the harm. Some researchers describe this as food addiction. In susceptible people, eating the food after a period of abstinence can produce a violent reaction not unlike that which is seen in response to narcotic drugs.

When these compounds are ingested regularly the adverse effects may become either more severe or more generalized to include other body tissues or systems, or the body may learn to adapt partially so that adverse symptoms are experienced when it does not get a dose of the allergen it craves. This is a type of withdrawal syndrome from the food addiction.

The situation is complicated by the fact that the response to the first intake may not have disappeared before the food is eaten again, with many other foods in between. Some of the commonly used foods like milk, eggs or wheat appear in disguise in many products, so that we are not always aware of eating them. The reactions that we can get to these foods may be allergy to one of the proteins or to some other compound. Because responses can occur in so many different ways, adverse reactions to food or other common environmental pollutants are difficult to recognize and characterize, but milk, wheat, eggs, yeast and food additives are common culprits.

Hyperactivity in childhood is considered to be the first phase of an environmental susceptibility reaction, but it takes an expert to distinguish between this condition and normal healthy exuberance. The problem may develop into the child becoming emotionally hypersensitive, tense, moody and argumentative as he or she grows older. Passionate hunger or thirst is a characteristic symptom of the condition.

With their constant demands for food and drink to satisfy their craving, children may also become obese.

If food allergy develops, so many diverse symptoms can be displayed that sufferers tend to be labelled as neurotic. Such a plethora of symptoms may be difficult to sort out, but they arise because the allergens are being ingested in varying amounts at different times, each producing its own reaction which may overlap with the reaction to another substance; meanwhile, the body is vainly trying to adapt to each new assault on the system. Few physiological disorders produce such a diverse range of symptoms, which often arise and disappear seemingly without cause – and this is another of the distinctive characteristics of food or environmental allergy. They may also appear to be associated with a particular food at one time but not at another, and they may produce their effect only if another allergen is present, and the system is already primed or weakened.

If you have symptoms like these, reaction to foreign compounds in your environment may be the cause. However, identifying and eliminating the source of your problem may be quite difficult. Much depends on how bad your response is. If it is only slight, you may decide to live with it. But for many people, reaction to their environment makes life intolerable, and anything that can be done to identify the cause and remedy the problem from a practical point of view should be encouraged, whether or not the treatment has a sound theoretical physiological basis.

The causes

First, we need to characterize those adverse reactions to food or other ingested substances which arise because we lack a specific enzyme necessary to process the substance. Into this category would fall intolerance of milk because of a lack of the enzyme needed to metabolize the galactose which is produced from the lactose found in the milk. An absence or inadequate production of the enzyme *aldolase* would make an individual intolerant of fruit because of the fructose it contains. Certain drugs can produce marked side effects in those patients who happen to be hypersensitive to them, that is, they don't have the enzymes necessary to detoxify the drugs in their bodies. The terms *intolerance* or *hypersensitivity* are appropriate in these cases.

The remaining cases of adverse reactions which are classified as *allergy* may indeed be correctly named, even in the restricted use of the word.

The production of classical allergic symptoms is associated with the release of chemicals like *histamine* and *serotonin* (*5-hydroxytryptamine*) within the body, particularly from sites called *mast cells*. These compounds are manufactured in the body from the amino acids *histidine* and *tryptophan* respectively, by simple reactions like the removal of carbon dioxide. Serotonin is also released in stress states, so that stress usually makes all forms of allergy worse.

Mast cells are a kind of white blood cell (or *leucocyte*) which are distributed throughout the body but which are found especially in connective tissue. This, as its name suggests, joins up one organ to another. It is found in the chest cavity and in the gut, where there are a number of organs that must be held in place, as well as in our limbs holding our bones together at the joints. Hence, these are the main sites of the mast cells.

When an antigen invades the body this generates the formation of immobilizing proteins (*immunoglobulins* or *antibodies*), which are made by other white blood cells. These attach on to the surface of the mast cells and when the system is exposed again to the antigen the mast cells are stimulated or ruptured to release histamine (particularly) into the surrounding tissues and blood stream. The lining or *epithelial* tissues are those which are most affected.

It has been suggested that this may also be the mechanism of environmental and food allergy: that proteins or other chemical molecules may react directly with our defence system or function as *haptens* – molecules which attach on to our natural proteins and alter their properties so much that they become antigenic. In this way, any substance could be made to behave as an antigen.

Why should this reaction occur? Has this process always existed but only recently been characterized, or is this a new type of disease? I suspect it may well be the latter. With a much more limited variety of foods in former times there should have been a greater chance of food allergy. With fewer variables to choose from it is likely that our ancestors would soon have associated a particular illness with a particular food. It should have been one of the earliest diseases to be identified, yet it was not so. Only now does this type of interaction seem to be emerging.

The human body was never intended to be exposed to the range of synthetic food additives and environmental pollutants to which it is now subjected. It may be that our bodies can tolerate a certain amount of these compounds, but then they respond adversely when the foreign substances are ingested in greater amounts or combined with one another, and our defence capability is exceeded. The extent of the adverse response depends initially on genetic susceptibility, and thereafter on earlier and current exposure.

In previous centuries our bodies were attacked by viruses and bacteria to which we have developed some defence mechanism through evolution. These have now been replaced by chemical intruders instead. There are many serious diseases like plague, smallpox, diphtheria, polio, tuberculosis and pneumonia which are now comparatively rare occurrences in developed countries, although many of them were rampant even half a century ago. In their place we have widespread minor ailments, like nervous, respiratory and digestive disorders; and major degenerative diseases like arteriosclerosis and cancer. Some of these can be correlated with an excess of sugar and fat, or a deficiency of fibre in the diet, but many of the illnesses have no definable organic cause and we cannot say at present what contribution the ingestion of toxins makes to these major or minor disorders.

One thing is certain: drugs, food additives and environmental pollutants are all toxic to our bodies in the sense that we derive no nutritional benefit from them and they have to be metabolized, rendered harmless and excreted. Logic tells us that none of us has an infinite capacity to cope with these chemicals and that sooner or later we may reach our limit for dealing with toxins, even though this tolerance capacity will vary greatly from one individual to another.

We can control our intake of drugs and food additives to some extent. More insidious is our bombardment with environmental pollutants. Not only are these largely beyond our immediate control, but also we may not even be aware of our exposure.

In recent years we have had several major chemical disasters brought to our attention: Love Canal (Niagara Falls), Flixborough (Yorkshire, UK), Minamata (Japan), Michigan (US), Seveso (Italy), Bhopal (India) and Karlskoga (Sweden) have all been the sites of serious chemical pollution that made international news. What we don't know, however, is the extent of the chemical contamination to which we may be exposed through the food we eat, the air we breathe, and the water we drink. We remain blissfully unaware of these until individual problems escalate into a regional epidemic. All we can do is to minimize our exposure as individuals and be ever aware of the potential hazards as a community. It seems quite feasible that the continual exposure to toxins to which we are subjected is straining our immune systems intolerably, so that normal food ingredients, which previously our bodies would have dealt with without any difficulty, are now posing problems.

For those who feel they may have this type of allergy, it is advisable to avoid the following common food additives:

1   All artificial colours (E102–160 in the European system).
2   Nitrite, nitrate, benzoate, gallate and sulphite preservatives (E210–229; E249, 250, 251; E310, 311, 312).
3   The flavouring monosodium glutamate (E621? – not yet assigned).

It should be noted, however, that some of the substances used as colourings, preservatives or emulsifiers are natural and harmless: for example, riboflavin (vitamin B2, E101); carotene (E160a); xanthophyll (E161); ascorbic acid (vitamin C, E300); tocopherol (vitamin E, E307–9); and lecithin (E322).

The cure

The only certain cure for food or environmental allergy is identification of the allergen and elimination of it from your diet or withdrawal of exposure. Identification isn't always easy: three- or four-day fasts followed by several weeks of eating foods one at a time is the sort of treatment that can be carried out effectively only in a clinic or hospital when you don't have a day's work to contend with.

In the normal home environment, you may still be able to fast for one or two days to help clear the system. Then go back on foods, if not one at a time, at least in small combinations: an early breakfast of one cereal with skimmed milk only; a couple of hours later, a boiled egg with toast and mineral water; and so on. You can still get an adequate quantity and variety of food to keep going, while at the same time giving yourself a good chance of tracking down an allergen. See if you can identify some food as consistently associated with your symptoms, though as already explained this may be difficult. Skin prick tests are not effective as a means of diagnosing food allergy.

It may be helpful for you to remember that wheat, milk and eggs are the most common food allergens, though of course they may not be yours. You may find that you are allergic to one whole *family* of foods, such as the nightshade group Solanaceae (potato, tomato, aubergine and peppers), or the Cruciferae brassicas (cabbage, cauliflower, broccoli and kale). However, the food family connection tends to be overemphasized by some clinical ecologists – you are almost certain to be more allergic to some members of a food family than others.

If yours is an environmental allergy, see if it improves when the central heating is on (allergy to mould spores?) or off (allergy to dust or gas fumes?). Is it better when you are out of doors or away from home? Try to associate your allergy with particular events or locations. If you have a seriously debilitating disease like arthritis or multiple sclerosis, you'll certainly need professional help to see if food or environmental allergy is the cause of your problem. Some clinical ecologists have achieved high success rates against even these diseases, but this is certainly not so in all cases.

Babies who are breast-fed for as long as possible seem to be less susceptible to allergy than those brought up on formula or cow's milk. This is because of the protection afforded by the *colostrum* and other ingredients in the mother's milk. Also, goat's milk, although more expensive than cow's milk, seems to provoke fewer allergy problems.

A new technique of treatment called 'neutralization' is being tried nowadays in Britain and America. It is highly controversial and there is no accepted scientific basis for it, but its practitioners claim a high success rate – over 90 per cent of those who visit one clinic in Surrey, England, for example, are able to lead a normal life. The idea is that patients are injected with lower and lower doses of allergen (not ever-increasing doses, as in desensitization), until the practitioner finds a dose just low enough *not* to provoke an allergic response. Periodic treatment with this dose then apparently gives immunity to the patients when they encounter the high dose of allergen in the environment in their normal everyday life. The immunity conferred is immediate – there is no time lag for a build-up effect.

Although many allergy specialists dismiss this whole concept, it is not at all unreasonable that high doses of an allergen will overload a vulnerable immune system, while a smaller dose might stimulate it to provide defence against much greater amounts of allergen on subsequent occasions. As we shall see in Chapter 23, this is the principle of homeopathic treatments, which have been used on many patients with great success for many years – indeed, for many more years than we have had orthodox medicine or allergy specialists!

I have met several patients with hay fever or asthma who maintain that if an attack is not bad enough to warrant medication, it often passes off by itself within a quarter- or half-hour. They then stay allergy-free for several days. If, on the other hand, they are forced to use high-dose medication, the condition will return within four to five hours and will continue to do so, with resulting dependence on the medication. Once again, it seems that the drugs, like the desensitization doses of allergen, swamp or inactivate the body's own defence mechanism, while the smaller doses used in 'neutralization therapy' or those which are met in slight natural exposure (or in homeopathy) stimulate the body's immune response. As antihistamine or sympathomimetic drugs almost always have unpleasant side effects, these cannot be considered a desirable solution. Even neutralization therapy has now been subjected to rigorous scientific study (including double-blind tests) and has been shown to be a valid form of treatment, whatever its mechanism, for both conventional and environmental allergy.

19

ALTERNATIVE MEDICINE:
an introduction

Despite all the advice now available about what we should do to cultivate our minds and train our bodies for perfect health, usually we don't quite make it. Either our willpower is not strong enough or the circumstances of our way of life – our diet, our job, our home situation – are such that we cannot achieve all of our objectives.

If things go wrong, the first course should be to consult the family physician as he should be in the best position to offer advice. If his recommendations don't work, you may then feel you want to try one of the alternative therapies.

These techniques are steadily gaining in popularity with the public, despite the lack of a rational basis for the treatment in many cases. This has gone along with a general disenchantment with the achievements of science and an increase of interest in the occult, astrology and psychic practices.

What is known as alternative medicine goes by many other names: it's also called natural, unorthodox, holistic or complementary medicine. It was in fact the original medical practice; it is orthodox medicine which is the newcomer. It wasn't until the seventeenth century that William Harvey put forward his ideas on the circulation of blood in the body, ideas which are at the root of modern medicine. Lister's antiseptics and Pasteur's germ theories are scarcely a century old; ether and chloroform made their appearance as anaesthetics at about the same time. Because its progress has been so rapid over the past two centuries, modern medicine has replaced natural healing as the established system. We shouldn't forget, however, that before then, so-called alternative medicine was all we had. Even today it is widely practised in Asia and Africa. It is only in the developed countries of the West that technological medicine dominates.

Slowly, and for the most part reluctantly, orthodox practitioners are admitting that alternative medicine does have something to offer. Much of the difficulty in acceptance of the methods of complementary medicine arises because the results cannot be measured in scientific terms. There are no standards against which their performance can be judged, other than success in particular cases. Because each patient is treated as an individual there are no groups of statistical data to interpret.

The greatest problem the alternative therapies have in being recognized as an intrinsic part of medicine arises from the use of unscientific concepts in attempting to explain the basis of some of the techniques. In other instances, accepted scientific ideas are applied in a totally inappropriate context. Some of the theories of alternative therapies actually defy established laws of science. Hence they cannot be accepted as rational explanations of how these practices produce their effects on the human body.

When we consider faith or religion we are dealing with communication between the mind or soul of the individual and his God or Christ or whoever the appropriate intermediary may be. It is entirely a personal matter for each one of us as an individual, even if we practise collectively.

When we are in the realms of science, however, we are dealing with phenomena which we must be able to perceive with our five senses. No longer can we talk in terms of belief or intuition. What we observe, everyone else must be able to observe. The results must be what the scientists call reproducible. This is where scientists encounter problems with some of the alternative therapies. Results are often not reproducible and tests are not carried out under standardized conditions. Thus, alternative medicine fails to meet scientific criteria both in theory and in practice.

In addition to what we can perceive with our five senses, there are events which most of us have experienced at some time that cannot be rationalized in this way. These arise from the powers we call intuition, or sixth sense, or psychic ability. It may be that these will be explained eventually in scientific terms of electromagnetic waves, though attempts to measure these so far have failed. For the present, however, we have to accept that these phenomena exist, whether we attribute them to as yet undetermined but perfectly logical 'scientific' forces, or to a higher divine being. Several of the alternative therapies involve these psychic phenomena.

Some studies suggest that nearly half the patients attending a doctor's surgery have no organic, physical ailment, only an affliction of the mind or spirit. We should not, therefore, reject out of hand those techniques which claim to effect diagnosis and treatment by communication with this spirit rather than with the physical body, just because we cannot understand or explain them.

The alternative practitioner sees this extrasensory force as providing the driving momentum for the body's chemical reactions. It is the force that faith healers invoke and that spiritualists commune with.

Perhaps the nearest we have come to a scientific demonstration of an unusual radiative force or energy was in the 1950s when the Russian investigators, Semyon and Valentina Kirlian, took special types of photographs of the fingertips of healers, of ordinary people, and of plants, under the influence of high-frequency alternating currents. The photographs they produced suggested that some sort of energy was radiated from the sources under these conditions, more from the healers and healthy plants.

It has been known for many years that atoms can be made to jump up to a higher energy (*excited*) state if they are subjected to an electric or magnetic field. When left to their own devices, with the field removed, these atoms fall back into the more stable lower energy (*ground*) state. The energy they absorb from the applied field in order to get to the higher energy state is given back out again. Whether or not this has anything to do with the Kirlian effect remains to be explored. But this is one instance where phenomena which were designated as irrational or psychic happenings have found a possible scientific interpretation.

For the present, if you choose alternative therapy you should be aware that it is essentially an act of faith. You are relying on the integrity and experience of the individual practitioners. Their skill is based on many centuries of practical experience – there is little theoretical scientific basis for what they do.

The alternative therapies now practised fall into two broad categories. There are those such as naturopathy, homeopathy, acupuncture, herbalism, and the Schuessler salts, all of which involve physical interaction with the body. In these cases, the effects of the treatment should be capable of scientific interpretation.

Then there are the techniques of the other group of practices, including healing by the laying on of hands, iridology and reflexology, sound and colour therapy, radiesthesia, radionics and psionic medicine, which involve spiritual or psychic communication. These methods cannot be rationalized and either have to be accepted as an act of faith or rejected.

The following chapters deal only with those alternative therapies which should have a logical scientific basis. The fact that their effects cannot always be explained in rational terms is no reason for the empirical practices themselves to be rejected. Their undoubted success in healing disease and their continued survival through thousands of years are reasons enough for them to merit serious consideration and more detailed investigation by scientific methods.

20

NATUROPATHY

This is a system of alternative medicine which treats patients by trying to find the root cause of their illnesses, and then endeavours to create conditions which allow the body to heal itself. Where there is an obvious cause, the disease is said to be organic; if the origin of the complaint is unknown, the illness is called a functional disease.

Naturopathy and drugs

Naturopathy and the other alternative therapies have progressed by astute observation of clinical conditions and their response to natural remedies. Despite a vast amount of basic research into causes of disease, conventional medical treatment has also evolved largely through clinical experiment. The explanation for the mode of action of a drug often emerges only after its successful use.

One of the fundamental tenets of conventional medicine, which goes back to the days of the Greek physician Hippocrates, is that if a doctor can do a patient no good, at least he should do him no harm. Unfortunately, some of the drugs most commonly prescribed today do not obey this principle. It is now a question of balancing the benefits of using the drug against the likelihood of possible side effects. For example, if aspirin is used frequently, particularly in an insoluble form, it is likely to produce bleeding from the wall of the gut. There is now a whole new branch of medicine (*iatrogenic medicine*) which is devoted to a study of those ailments caused by the administration of drugs.

For this reason, naturopaths try to stimulate the body's own defence and healing mechanisms by natural agents rather than prescribe unnatural and artificial pharmacological preparations. Naturopathic treatment therefore does not produce side effects.

Naturopathy as holistic medicine

If a patient complains of a pain, the cause may be physical, mental or biochemical. A pain in the left arm, for example, may be due to a broken bone, pulled muscle, sprained tendon, inflammation of the joints (arthritis), or a symptom of heart disease. It all depends on the location, frequency, and nature of the pain. It is least likely to be due to a biochemical or emotional disturbance, although recent research suggests that arthritis may arise in just that way, through a biochemical imbalance.

On the other hand, a pain in the stomach may indicate an ulcer, but is much more likely to be indigestion resulting from a biochemical or emotional problem. Headaches are also most likely to arise from a similar cause. In both cases the problem is less likely to be physical in origin.

It is in these latter cases that naturopathy comes into its own. Instead of merely prescribing an antacid or a painkiller, the naturopath will try to identify the fundamental problem producing the symptom. Perhaps the patient's job is such that he eats poorly balanced meals too fast, or perhaps he works daily in artificial light or in a noisy environment. He may be under excessive stress from the home or work environment.

The naturopath will look beyond the symptoms, beyond even the direct cause of the symptoms, to the fundamental problem. Whether or not it is easily soluble is another matter. The resolution may demand a change of job or of home location. It is quite often some aspect of the patient's lifestyle which produces the symptoms of illness.

Naturopathy requires far greater understanding of the patient than is practicable in conventional medicine. The amount of time required to achieve such understanding is simply not available in current medical practice. Nor does every doctor subscribe to the philosophy that such fundamental understanding is necessary.

We may get, for example, a diagnosis of a skin disease or a nervous disorder if we see our family doctor; but the naturopath will view the same complaint as a whole-body malfunction which manifests itself with symptoms in the skin or nerves. The conventional practitioner sees the problem as a disorder of a specific system or organ.

Naturopathy is essentially a practice of holistic medicine – treating the whole person in his or her environment. Holistic medicine, involving the mind and spirit (or soul, or psyche, or whatever you want to call it) together with physical treatment, is currently enjoying a renaissance in the West even with conventional practitioners, but the idea is not new. The Indians especially have had their ayurvedic medicine for centuries. The word *ayurveda* is a Sanskrit word meaning 'knowledge of life', and the philosophy encompasses the inseparability of mind, body and soul. Although many orthodox doctors will not embrace this idea, there are others who use it more and more in their practice, whether or not they overtly acknowledge it as holistic medicine.

The healing force

Naturopaths and many other alternative practitioners believe that the body possesses an internal energy beyond that which we can measure scientifically and which is generated by the mind or soul. It is this energy that is harnessed for self-healing. This idea goes back thousands of years to the earliest Oriental physicians. The Chinese call this energy *chi* (or *ch'i*); the Japanese know it as *ki*; Hindu philosophers and physicians call it *prana*. It is equivalent to Wilhelm Reich's 'orgone energy', and homeopaths describe it as 'the vital force'. Alexander Lowen's psychotherapeutic techniques of self-healing, developed in the 1950s and using what he calls 'Bioenergetics', employ the same principle. This concept is also the essence of Dr Vernon Coleman's 'Bodypower'.

The body unquestionably has great reserves of self-healing (and self-destruction!). This is acknowledged by orthodox as well as alternative medical practitioners. If we think ourselves well we can often achieve 'spontaneous remission' of an illness. Dr Alec Forbes has produced some remarkable results in recent years using this philosophy to treat cancer patients in Bristol, Avon, with a combination of psychological and nutritional therapy.

This internal healing force which the body possesses is also described, as mentioned above, as 'the vital force', a term which implies a force or energy associated with life (since it comes from the Latin word *vitalis*, meaning 'life'). This is where one of the conceptual problems arises, since all objects, organic and inorganic, plants and animals as well as natural inanimate substances, are all believed to possess 'a vital force'.

The nature of this force or energy in humans may eventually be given some scientific interpretation. There are others who would consider it extracorporeal and bestowed by God. Whatever the point of view, to endow inanimate objects with the same property would seem to transgress both scientific and religious principles.

Naturopathy and science

There is certainly nothing unscientific about the natural and holistic approach to disease therapy, though conventional practitioners may regard it as inadequate for treating anything but the most trivial disorders. Few would accept yet that it has any relevance in the treatment of cancer. There are, however, some naturopathic concepts which would be unacceptable to most conventional scientists.

Disease is regarded by naturopaths as originating within the body, not invading it from outside. They accept that when we are ill bacteria or viruses may be seen in the blood stream or tissues. These, it is held, are released or generated from an internal source by the illness. Microbes are thus regarded as the result rather than the cause of disease, and hence naturopaths do not believe in the use of antibiotics or other drugs for killing germs.

When symptoms of disease appear, they are viewed by naturopaths as a manifestation of the body's healing processes and therefore not usually something to be quenched. It is interesting to note that some orthodox practitioners are now reluctant to prescribe drugs just for the relief of symptoms, provided they are not unbearable or life-threatening. Orthodox doctors would regard some symptoms as a sign of disorder and others as an indication of healing.

Naturopaths describe the flare-up of symptoms as 'healing crises'. Naturopathic (and homeopathic) treatments often promote or even provoke these healing crises rather than alleviate them, as a method of stimulating the body's own defence mechanisms.

The extent to which a naturopathic practitioner will try to provoke healing crises depends on the individual's energy reserves or 'vitality'. This individual quality is not precisely defined other than as an ability to overcome disease; nor is there any method of quantifying it – exactly how much vitality does each person have? This is not just an academic question. The naturopath must assess the individual's ability to withstand the healing crises in order to effect the cure.

The naturopathic explanation of epidemics is not that they are carried by the spread of an organism, but rather that a lot of people living under similar environmental conditions fall prey to one of their internal viruses or bacteria at the same time. Since the very foundation of naturopathy is the concept of individuality, the idea that so many people should be similar enough to fall prey to the same microbe at the same time doesn't seem to be consistent.

Practitioners of both philosophies, orthodox and unorthodox, would agree that for a person to become ill two factors are required: the agent causing the illness, and the susceptibility of the individual. This susceptibility may either be inherited or acquired as a result of malnutrition or environmental influences. All would agree that the higher a person's vitality or stamina or fitness, the better they are able to avoid or to recover from disease.

It is difficult to get a scientific assessment of the effectiveness of naturopathy overall for a number of reasons. The whole philosophy of treatment is to regard each person as an individual. The standard scientific practices of matched controls and double-blind tests are therefore impossible and no statistical trends can ever be established. Furthermore, because of the whole-body approach, naturopathic treatment almost always involves more than one prescription for health. A scientific study would need to assess the effects of one specific treatment at a time.

Naturopathy is tantamount to a philosophy, a way of life. The naturopath advocates abstinence from tea, coffee, alcohol, smoking, drugs, refined foods and those which contain additives, in addition to personal recommendations for each individual. The lifestyle prescribed can hardly fail to be an improvement on what most of us actually practise. No wonder many people get better after visiting a naturopath!

Naturopathic principles make a great contribution to health in several ways: by seeking out the causes of disease rather than treating symptoms; by advocating fresh air, exercise and wholesome natural foods; and by recognizing the contributions to our well-being which are made by the mind and spirit. These concepts may be even more successful in the prevention of disease than in their cure.

SUPPLEMENTARY TECHNIQUES

There are many auxiliary techniques which naturopaths employ for diagnosis and treatment.

Osteopathy is a technique of manipulative treatment. It was devised by Andrew T. Still, who founded the American School of Osteopathy in 1892. Still's doctrine, first proposed in 1874, was that all diseases arise from lesions of the joints and that these in turn are caused by faulty blood supply. The purpose of manipulation is to correct this.

Chiropractic is a closely related philosophy of treatment by manipulation founded by a Canadian physician, Daniel D. Palmer, in 1895. Palmer's idea was that disease was caused by inadequate nerve supply to the muscles and other organs. Great emphasis is placed on spinal manipulation in chiropractic since the spine is the centre of nervous impulses in the body.

Osteopathy and chiropractic are now recognized as effective therapeutic techniques even by the orthodox medical establishment.

Iridology involves a study of the iris, the coloured portion at the front of the eyeball, for diagnosis. Different regions of the iris are taken to represent various systems or organs of the body, and the condition of the organ is supposed to be reflected in the condition of the corresponding tiny portion of the iris. Most iridologists will take a picture of the eye so that they can study the iris in detail when the patient isn't available.

Reflexology uses a complementary idea for diagnosis and treatment in which each part of the foot is said to be connected by nerves to a remote part of the body. By pressing on the foot in each place in turn, the reflexologist assesses the state of health of the various organs, since disorder in the organ is indicated by tenderness in the foot. Massage of the foot, it is claimed, produces stimulation of the organ.

There is no physiological basis for either iridology or reflexology. There are no direct nerve connections between the organs of the body and either the iris or the foot. The only lines of communication are through the central nervous system (brain and spinal cord) or via the blood stream. Furthermore, there are direct nervous connections between the brain and all the organs and systems in our body – they could not function otherwise. But disorder in these organs does not usually show up as a disorder in the brain. That organ malfunction should show up in the eye or foot therefore has no rational scientific foundation.

Certain types of systemic disease are visible in the retina, however. You may be surprised to have your optician tell you that you have circulation problems when you get your eyes tested, but the state of the blood vessels at the back of the eye is a good indication of their condition elsewhere in the body. This type of information can be derived for only a few specific disorders and the condition of the retina as a whole is taken into account. The iris is bathed in fluid through which nutrients or toxins can move freely. It is therefore hard to envisage that minute adjacent portions of the iris should differ so fundamentally as to indicate health or disease of quite unconnected organs.

Radiesthesia, radionics and psionic medicine   all use psychic interaction between patient and practitioner to influence the behaviour of a pendulum as a means of diagnosis. The concept is similar to that used in water divining.

Sound and colour therapy   both utilize the restorative effects of sound or light of a particular frequency for treatment. All radiation has a specific energy associated with it which is directly proportional to the frequency. High-frequency (or short-wavelength) blue light has a higher energy than the lower-frequency (longer-wavelength) red colours. A high-pitched sound has a higher energy than a low rumble. It has been shown scientifically that people do respond differently to radiation of different energies. Some are greatly disturbed by the low-frequency sound emitted by domestic appliances, for example. Most of us find some colours soothing, others more disturbing. It cannot be said, however, that there is any scientific rationale behind either sound or colour therapy.

Megavitamin therapy   is a technique developed a few decades ago by several pioneer practitioners who were all orthodox physicians. It entails treating illness by the use of vitamins in high doses. Vitamin B for mental disturbance was the first to be used in this way. H. M. Clerkley published a scientific paper in 1939 in the *Journal of the American Medical Association* on the use of niacin for treating psychiatric disturbance, while Abram Hoffer and Humphrey Osmond (unaware of Clerkley's work) treated schizophrenia with niacin in the 1950s.

Linus Pauling has probably become more famous in the eyes of the general public for his advocacy of high doses of vitamin C than for the outstanding work on chemical structures which won him a Nobel Prize. Pauling maintains that vitamin C in gram amounts daily wards off colds and respiratory tract infections, and perhaps many other ailments too. Pauling coined the term 'orthomolecular medicine' for this type of therapy, which he defined in the late 1960s as 'the preservation of good health and the treatment of disease by varying the concentrations in the human body of substances that are normally present and required for health'. Whatever the merits of the vitamin C recommendations, most of us would be much happier if our ills could be treated, cured or, even better, prevented by natural body compounds, rather than having our symptoms treated after the disease has developed with a medicine cabinet full of potentially toxic drugs.

The distinction between megavitamin therapy and orthomolecular medicine is that the advocates of the former generally recommend massive doses of almost all mineral and vitamin nutrients in the belief that the body will reject what it doesn't require. Practitioners of orthomolecular medicine are much more selective as to which minerals and vitamins they suggest for increased intake. Their aim is to tailor the prescription for each individual.

Negative ion therapy, considered in detail on its own in Chapter 25, should also be listed here as a supplementary naturopathic treatment.

All of these techniques, like naturopathy, are non-invasive; there are no needles or injections, and no synthetic drugs of any kind are used.

21

SCHUESSLER SALTS

The Schuessler salts, also called biochemic, tissue or cell salts, are a group of twelve inorganic compounds which are used to treat a variety of ailments. All except one (silica) are salts in the chemical sense of the word (more will be said about that later). They are listed below, with their numbers, abbreviated names (which are based on the old Latin names of the elements) and full chemical names:

1	Calc Fluor	calcium fluoride
2	Calc Phos	calcium phosphate
3	Calc Sulph	calcium sulphate
4	Ferr Phos	iron phosphate
5	Kali Mur	potassium chloride
6	Kali Phos	potassium phosphate
7	Kali Sulph	potassium sulphate
8	Mag Phos	magnesium phosphate
9	Nat Mur	sodium chloride
10	Nat Phos	sodium phosphate
11	Nat Sulph	sodium sulphate
12	Silica	silicon dioxide

The Schuessler salts are prescribed widely by naturopaths and homeopaths as a part of their courses of treatment, though these compounds are in a class by themselves: they are not truly naturopathic or homeopathic remedies. Naturopaths address themselves to causes of disease, whereas the Schuessler salts are used to treat symptoms. Homeopaths use substances foreign to the body to generate symptoms, whereas the Schuessler salts are supposed to suppress symptoms and, with the exception of No. 12, are all substances found naturally in the body. They are, however, prepared by the homeopathic principle of successive dilution (*attenuation*).

As discussed in Chapter 27, all the constituents of the active principles of Schuessler salts are natural components of cells: potassium and phosphate, with much smaller concentrations of magnesium and sulphate, are found in the fluid inside the cell; sodium and chloride in the fluid outside the cell; calcium in bone cells; and iron in red blood cells. The twelfth Schuessler salt contains silicon, as in chips. At the present time, more than a century after Schuessler, there is no evidence that this is an essential nutrient in humans.

The Schuessler salts are one of the less convincing forms of alternative therapy, mainly for two reasons.

When Dr William H. Schuessler did his work in Germany in the middle of the last century, a substance like sodium chloride (common salt) was thought to be a single indivisible chemical entity. It wasn't until the 1880s that a Swedish chemist called Arrhenius suggested that sodium chloride and all other chemical salts in fact split up into two parts, the sodium part and the chloride part, just as soon as they are put in water. These two parts carry positive and negative charges respectively and are called *ions*. The same would be true for all of the cell salts, except No. 12. Silica is not a salt; it is an acidic oxide similar, in some ways, to carbon dioxide: both are only sparingly soluble in water.

From the work of chemists in the first part of this century more information has now come to light about salts. We now know that sodium chloride, for example, is made up of sodium ions and chloride ions just as soon as it is formed. There is no sodium (metal) or chlorine (gas) as such in common salt. We don't even have to wait for salts to be dissolved in water to get ions. All salts are made up of ions as they are formed: they cannot be made any other way. Putting them in water allows the ions to drift apart from each other so that they have a more or less independent existence (see Figure 5).

Thus the sodium ion in Nat Mur is identical in every respect to the sodium ion in Nat Sulph, and the chloride in Nat Mur is identical in every respect to the chloride in Kali Mur. They cannot be different. Yet the health-giving properties ascribed to the three sodium salts are significantly different. So are those of the three potassium salts, and so on. With inorganic 'compounds', the properties of mixtures are usually the sum of the properties of the individual components of the mixture. (With organic compounds, the properties of mixtures can be very different from those of the components – what is called *synergism*.)

Similarly, there cannot possibly be any difference between a combination of, say, Nat Mur with Kali Sulph, and Nat Sulph with Kali Mur. In both cases we have a combination not of two different compounds but of four identical ions: sodium, potassium, chloride and sulphate.

Thus we should expect that Nat Mur would have some properties in common with Nat Sulph and Nat Phos, since they all contain sodium ions. Similarly with all the potassium salts and all the different calcium salts. Yet there is little or no evidence of this in the literature which

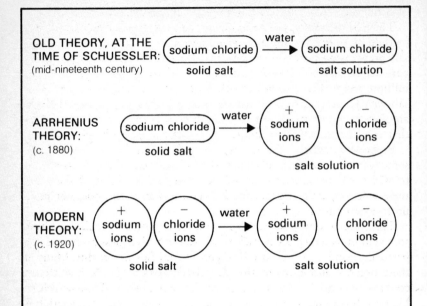

OLD THEORY, AT THE TIME OF SCHUESSLER: (mid-nineteenth century)

sodium chloride — water → sodium chloride

solid salt   salt solution

ARRHENIUS THEORY: (c. 1880)

sodium chloride — water → + sodium ions   − chloride ions

solid salt   salt solution

MODERN THEORY: (c. 1920)

+ sodium ions   − chloride ions — water → + sodium ions   − chloride ions

solid salt   salt solution

Figure 5 The ionic theory. The figure shows how our ideas about salt formation have evolved over the years

accompanies these Schuessler salts.

It is appropriate to note here also that the fluoride in Calc Fluor tablets cannot be any different from the natural or artificial fluoride in drinking water, except that the amount in the Schuessler salt tablets is so minute. You will probably take in more fluoride from your toothpaste or morning tea than you are ever likely to get out of the Schuessler tablets.

This brings us to the second objection to the likely effectiveness of these Schuessler salt tablets as a therapeutic remedy: the minute amount of active ingredient present. There are in the human body, as we have seen, many hormones and nutrients which are present only in microgram amounts. If a person is deficient in one of these substances, addition of this small quantity to the diet, or a few micrograms injected into the blood stream, may indeed produce a marked effect.

When, however, an individual has a normal daily intake of from 1 to 2 g of sodium (mostly as salt, sodium chloride) and about double that amount of potassium, the few millionths of a gram present in each dose of Schuessler salts cannot possibly have any influence.

These Schuessler salts, like homeopathic remedies, are prepared by the method of *attenuation* or successive dilution. The strength of Schuessler salt preparation normally sold in health food shops is x6, that is, one part active ingredient in 10^6 (one million) parts of tablet. Only one millionth part therefore of each of those tiny white tablets is really the salt we pay for. The rest is lactose filler. When we compare that with the amount of salt that we sprinkle on our chips, for example, we can see that the amount extra in the Schuessler tablets is negligible.

Proponents of this treatment maintain that the salt in the tablets is in some way made 'accessible' by the process of grinding down (*trituration*) to which the components are subjected, an accessibility which is not there when we eat salt in our food. Again, this argument does not stand up to examination.

There are certainly some large, complex organic molecules and even some vitamins which are not accessible to the body unless presented in a particular form or unless specific digestive enzymes are present. Many of these organic nutrients are also destroyed (denatured or degraded) by cooking or other food processing. But ions are almost indestructible in biological systems. Once they are put into water, they are available. Grinding cannot introduce any difference between the sodium chloride of Nat Mur tablets and the sodium chloride in the commercial salt used in cooking.

If Schuessler tablets produce any beneficial effects at all – and the evidence for this is far from convincing – these will almost certainly come from the self-healing principle described previously (Chapter 20) or from the lactose which makes up 99.9999 per cent of every tablet. Lactose is sugar. Just as we feel a lift from eating a bar of chocolate, so we will almost certainly get a similar sense of uplift from the Schuessler salt tablets, especially if they are taken three times a day as recommended. There must be many more effective and less expensive forms of therapy.

22

HERBALISM

Herbalism is a system of alternative medicine in which drugs are extracted from natural plant sources instead of being manufactured. For thousands of years Man has sought out certain plants to cure his ills. Even today, in many parts of Asia and Africa herbal medicine is the method of treatment used in everyday therapy. In the Western world it is practised in Britain probably more than in any other country, partly because of the laws concerning the operation of practitioners, and partly because of the country's long traditional use of herbalism which the New World does not have.

Herbal preparations differ from the drugs of the pharmaceutical industry in several important ways, though they do have at least one thing in common. Let's look at the differences first:

1 Sometimes a herbalist will use only one specific plant to remedy an illness. Usually, however, herbal preparations are mixtures. In pharmacy, drugs used to be dispensed which were also mixtures of several ingredients, but nowadays the majority of prescription drugs are single compounds.

With inorganic compounds, the reactions and bodily effects of a mixture are likely to be the sum of the effects of the component parts (see page 131). When we look at the physiological properties of organic compounds like those in herbal extracts, this is frequently not the case. We often find that they interfere with one another when they are used together (an effect known as *synergism*). A mixture may well have a greater or lesser effect, and occasionally a completely different one, from that of the individual compounds. The success of herbal preparations therefore owes little to science and a great deal to heritage and the experience of the practitioner.

2 Herbalist preparations are all extracted from natural plant sources. The pharmaceutical industry now makes almost all of its drugs synthetically by a series of chemical reactions, though it may get the starting material from a natural source.

As the lines of synthetic investigation become ever more exploited, drug companies are now themselves taking an interest in isolating active principles from plant sources, or seeing if they can modify or improve on a potent plant ingredient to retain the therapeutic value without undesirable side effects.

3   The concentration of an active ingredient in a plant varies greatly. It depends on the length of time the plant has been growing, the climate and seasonal weather in that region, the geological nature and past history of the soil in which the plant is grown, and even the time of day at which the plant is picked.

All the chemical substances in a plant have to be synthesized or accumulated from the soil or from the air. There is only so much nutrient in any patch of soil. No natural soil is ever likely to have every nutrient the plant requires unless it has been specifically prepared.

Consequently, although the composition and general level of concentration of natural products in a plant species will be the same from one specimen to another, there are considerable variations in both the quantity and nature of components in any plant. This variation is carried through to many of the herbal preparations.

Variation in composition to any significant degree is rare in pharmaceutical drugs. Conditions of manufacture are rigorously controlled so that the amount of active ingredient from one tablet to the next, or from one batch of medicine to the next, is constant. That same degree of control is necessary also to exclude contamination.

With regard to contamination, one further point may be mentioned. Herbal remedies are prepared when required and tend to be used in a relatively short period of time thereafter. Conventional drugs are mass-produced and stored until needed, perhaps already several months after manufacture.

There does seem to be a tendency for patients to hoard such drugs for considerable periods of time, possibly because of the cost of them, or perhaps because they don't want to be thought of as a hypochondriac by the family doctor. Whatever the reason, many prescription drugs are used long after the date intended. Not only may the active ingredient have deteriorated by this time, and thus be less effective, but also other end-products may have been formed by the effects of heating by air temperature or radiators, or through attack by moisture. The expiry dates on drugs should, therefore, always be heeded.

So much for the differences between herbal and conventional drug preparations. One property that the two classes of medication have in common is that the substances administered are foreign to the body. They are not compounds which are either nutrients or intermediates in the body's chemistry. That is the definition of a drug: a compound foreign to the body which produces a physiological effect. Herbal medicines are still drugs!

Treatment of an ailment by an experienced herbalist has much to offer, though there is no reason scientifically why the treatment should be more or less effective than the corresponding drugs prescribed by a competent orthodox physician. It is largely a matter of personal choice. The problem is mainly one of establishing the qualifications of the herbalist.

Herbalists, like doctors, do treat symptoms. On the other hand, like naturopaths, herbalists will also try to identify causes of disorders in a way that time and training rarely permit the family physician to do. Most consultations with herbalists and naturopaths take half-an-hour or more; diagnosis and prescription in the doctor's surgery usually occupies five minutes or less. Whereas the natural therapist tends to look more widely for causes of illness, the conventional doctor tends to concentrate on the immediate problem.

On probing more deeply the systemic disorder, the herbalist will use plant preparations to try to stimulate the body's own defence mechanisms, hoping to alleviate the symptoms of disorder in the process. Once again, an assessment of lifestyle in order to correct any fundamental problem is an integral part of herbalist treatment, as in naturopathy.

Some herbalist treatments are well known and are available in any health product store; they are intended to be used without medical supervision. Others most definitely require careful monitoring. Let's look at some examples.

If a patient has indigestion, a herbalist may well recommend extract of pawpaw or pineapple, which both contain the protein-digesting enzyme *papain*. Tablets of papain are prepared by several different companies which specialize in natural remedies. This enzyme is effective only in digesting proteins. Some firms produce extracts intended to stimulate the growth of natural gut bacteria to help in digestion.

Extract of evening primrose (*Oenothera biennis*) is used as a sedative, for treating hypertension (and thus reducing the risk of heart attacks), and for pre-menstrual tension. The active ingredient is the unsaturated lipid *linolenic acid* (also known as GLA).

Ginseng (*Panax sp.*) has long been regarded in the East as a general tonic or stimulant. Modern research has isolated from the root of this plant one compound which reduces blood sugar and others that stimulate the heart and nervous sytem.

The heart-stimulating properties of the foxglove (*Digitalis purpurea*) have been known for centuries. The active ingredients from *Digitalis sp.* (*digitoxin, digoxin* and *gitoxin*) are used by doctors, and the plant extracts themselves by herbalists, for the treatment of irregularities in the heart beat (*cardiac arrhythmia*).

For nasal congestion, health stores sell a blend of essential oils which includes eucalyptus, menthol, peppermint, wintergreen, juniper and cajuput, with a dash of cloves. In most cases it is just as effective as the mixture prescribed by physicians, which also contains aromatic essential oils.

These are just a few common instances of the use of plant extracts for the treatment of disorders by both conventional and alternative practitioners.

There are now many books on the subject of herbalism, of varying degrees of complexity. As the techniques have been practised since long before the Middle Ages, such books have been published since the invention of printing, but it was the seventeenth-century herbalist Nicholas Culpeper who wrote what is still regarded as one of the most authoritative books on the subject in the English language, *A Physicall Directory* (1649).

Only a few per cent of the many thousands of known plant species have so far been investigated for their medicinal properties. Each country naturally tends to use its own local plants, and everyone could benefit from an exchange of information between Western herbalists, Chinese country doctors and African tribal medicine men. Almost certainly, many more herbal preparations will be used all over the world in the years ahead, by both practising herbalists and conventional pharmacologists.

BACH REMEDIES

These are a specific kind of herbal preparation, developed by Edward Bach and first proposed in detail in his book *The Twelve Healers*, which was published in 1933. Born in 1880, Bach had a traditional medical training and practised for a time in Harley Street, London, but he abandoned orthodox medicine for a system of healing which he felt was more in harmony with nature.

Bach suggested that all illness is essentially emotional. He devised his system of aqueous plant extracts, originally twelve in number but later thirty-eight in all, to treat seven groups of emotional problems: fear, uncertainty, apathy, loneliness, hypersensitivity, despair and neurosis.

Bach treated his patients for these emotional conditions rather than for the physical symptoms which, he maintained, were merely the manifestation of the underlying psychological disturbance.

The remedies are not homeopathic – they do not provoke symptoms of disease. Nor are they prepared in various potencies. Their healing power is allegedly that of the plant life force.

Scientists today would regard these treatments, like other forms of herbalism, as owing their success, if any, to chemical substances within the plant, just like any other drugs. It should be mentioned, however, that some analyses have failed to find any plant compounds in the aqueous extracts prepared. The self-healing effect mentioned previously cannot be ruled out in some cases of successful treatment.

Dr Bach lived near Wallingford, Oxfordshire, where the Bach Centre is still located; he died in 1936.

AROMATHERAPY

This is a variation of herbalism in which aromatic or essential oils from plants are inhaled, taken internally like any other drug, or massaged into the skin.

The use of menthol for bronchial congestion; eucalyptus for sore throats (as an *antiseptic*); oil of wintergreen, peppermint or spearmint to aid digestion (as a *carminative*); witch hazel extract for rheumatism (as an *anti-inflammatory* agent); and liquorice for coughs and asthma, to soothe the airways (as a *demulcent*) and loosen phlegm (as an *expectorant*) are just a few common examples of aromatherapy in practice.

23
HOMEOPATHY

The origins of homeopathy

The foundation of this technique was first laid by the German physician Samuel Hahnemann, who was born in Meissen in 1755. He studied medicine in Leipzig and Vienna, and after qualification he settled and practised in Leipzig. It was there, beginning in 1790, that he undertook the studies which eventually led to the publication in 1810 of his seminal work *The Organon of Rational Healing*. This contained an exposition of his theories and a statement of the two principles on which homeopathy is based – namely, that 'like cures like' and that 'the actions of drugs are potentiated by dilution'.

Both of the specific deductions which Hahnemann extended to provide these two generalizations are, in fact, erroneous. For the first, he found that when he took quinine, which was used to treat malaria, it induced a malaria fit in him. According to some accounts, he had already suffered from malaria previously, in which case there need not have been any direct association between the fit and the self-administered quinine. Even if we leave this possibility aside, it would have to be said that headaches, nausea, vomiting, diarrhoea and fever accompany many illnesses, including malaria. They are also the most frequent symptoms of drug poisoning. They are an indication of the body's attempt to rid itself of toxins, bacterial or chemical, and they do not imply any connection between drug and disease, beyond the fact that they are both foreign to the body. It is hardly surprising, therefore, that Hahnemann found in many cases that drugs and diseases produced similar symptoms. His error was in concluding that the drug and symptoms were in some way related.

The dilution idea was generated from treatments he applied using mercury. These were indeed made more effective during the dilution process, though not because of the dilution itself but because the mercury was converted during the procedure to more potent oxides of the metal, which enhanced the pharmacological effects.

Hahnemann's greatest contribution to medicine was probably his introduction of the concept of clinical pharmacology – the testing of the effects of drugs on healthy individuals. This is one of the cornerstones of modern pharmaceutical practice. (The other is carrying out tests on animals and inferring that the drugs will have a similar effect on humans.)

Hahnemann's homeopathic drugs (the term is taken from the Latin words for 'like the disease') produced the same symptoms in healthy people as his sick patients had acquired from the disease. Conventional medicine was distinguished as allopathy (from the Latin words for 'different from the disease'): here, drugs are used primarily to eliminate symptoms.

Homeopathic preparations

The drugs prescribed by homeopaths are usually herbal in nature. Less common are the salts of heavy metals like gold, mercury and arsenic. Least used are biological extracts of sputum bacteria which are prepared from infected patients.

In the preparation of homeopathic drugs, the compound is diluted one part in ten parts (occasionally, one in a hundred parts) of water or lactose. The resulting one-tenth dilution is denoted by x1. This is further diluted one part in ten to give strength x2, and so on. A strength of x6, which is one of the most commonly used, represents one part of active ingredient in 10^6 (one million) parts of preparation. This process is known as *potentiation*. The grinding up of the active ingredient (*trituration*) and shaking with dilutant (*succussion* or *succussation*) are essential parts of the preparation.

Mode of action: practical considerations

In many cases homeopathic remedies do undoubtedly work; in others, they don't. How is the effect achieved when it is successful?

The mind is an extremely powerful controlling influence, for good or ill, on conditions of the body. People believing themselves to be ill, or cured of some disease, do indeed get sick, or better, on occasions without physical intervention. This self-healing explanation as a rationalization of the effectiveness of homeopathic remedies in some cases cannot be ignored. This effect is frequently met in administration of conventional medicines also. Studies suggest that self-healing or spontaneous remission achieved in this way may account for the cure in as many as one-third of all patients, by either technique. There have been too many successful homeopathic treatments under controlled conditions, however, for this explanation to hold good in all cases, so we must look for other possibilities.

It is well established that small quantities of a drug can stimulate the body's own defence mechanisms against disease where a large dose of the same drug overwhelms them: we have many effective self-correcting systems in our bodies. This principle is used in orthodox pharmacology, in traditional herbalism, and in desensitizing allergy sufferers by giving them ever-increasing doses of allergen. Even vaccination employs a somewhat similar concept, using dead germs (as in polio) or biologically similar germs (as in cowpox for smallpox) to stimulate the body's own defence agents (*antibodies*). These same principles of action undoubtedly hold for successful homeopathic remedies.

If either physically or mentally initiated self-healing each produced a cure in just 25 per cent of the people treated homeopathically, we would have perfectly feasible explanations for the success rate of homeopathic therapy.

One reason why conventional drugs sometimes 'cure' a disease where homeopathy fails is that synthetic drugs are so much stronger and are specifically designed to alleviate symptoms. Homeopathic drugs rarely do this; they aim to stimulate the body to correct itself, and where they fail, they may simply not be strong enough. Because of the low doses of active ingredients that they contain, homeopathic drugs rarely produce any side effect.

Why should homeopathic remedies work if Schuessler salts do not? First, homeopathic preparations are often given in doses stronger than x6, the usual Schuessler salt potency, which increases the amount of active ingredient perhaps one thousand-fold over that in the Schuessler salts. Second, and much more importantly, homeopathic treatments always involve compounds which are foreign to the body. All Schuessler salts (except silica) contain millionths of a gram of salts found in gram quantities in the body.

Although they are not intended to provoke symptoms of disease in healthy individuals, Schuessler salts are sometimes used by homeopaths for treatment, though for this and the reasons just mentioned, they cannot be regarded as homeopathic compounds.

Homeopathy should, in principle, be able to treat any illness that naturopathy, herbalism or conventional drug therapy can treat, provided the drugs used are strong enough. It all depends on the skill of the practitioner. Illnesses demanding physical intervention in the body – manipulation or surgery – cannot be treated by homeopaths.

Mode of action: theoretical considerations

From a theoretical point of view, when homeopathy succeeds as a treatment it probably does so for perfectly rational scientific reasons. There is no need to invoke non-scientific forces as an explanation since, as indicated above, our existing knowledge explains the effect adequately. Certainly, some of the theoretical interpretations offered by homeopaths do not withstand scientific scrutiny. Let's take a look at some of these now.

Homeopaths maintain that active ingredients dissolved in water in some way imprint themselves on the water molecules and that this imprint remains even if the original substance is removed. Some homeopathic preparations are so weak that the probability of finding even one molecule of active ingredient remaining in the medication is extremely small. Now, water molecules are in a state of continuous movement (known as Brownian Motion) and never stay for any significant time in any one position or pattern: this is what makes water a liquid. So the possibility of a solute pattern in the liquid is untenable.

As for some characteristic energy being transferred from active principle to water: there are only certain forms that energy can assume and any energy transmitted into the water would become kinetic energy – energy of movement of the water molecules – which would not give the water any distinctive properties other than to raise its temperature by an infinitesimal amount.

Another idea put forward by homeopaths is that the process of grinding down the active principle with lactose increases the energy of the mixture to form energy-rich crystal lattices according to the principles of crystal field theory. But powders are not single crystal lattices; they are an aggregate of millions of individual crystals, and the energy supplied in grinding goes to break up the crystals into smaller fragments and not to provide any binding or crystal energy.

Each crystal lattice has a well-defined energy which is characteristic of the atoms in the lattice. It is physically impossible to put active ingredients inside a lactose crystal lattice or to change its energy by grinding. It is sometimes stated that the doping of semiconductors with impurities is an analogous process, but in fact it is totally different. Semiconductors are prepared by the *chemical* addition of impurities: these do form part of the crystal structure and they do alter the properties of the pure material.

Wave-particle duality is another widely accepted and impressive-sounding scientific concept which is invoked to explain the activity of homeopathic remedies. The solid active principle owes its healing effect, it is claimed, to the wave energy associated with it. The wave-particle theory was put forward in 1924 by the French scientist Louis de Broglie. In essence, the theory states that particles have a wave energy associated with them and can behave sometimes as if they were solid particles and sometimes as if they were packets of wave energy.

This idea was proposed to account for the behaviour of particles of electricity (*electrons*) and has since been shown to be relevant for other sub-atomic particles. In the body it could apply only to the two types of sub-atomic particles found there (*electrons* and *protons*). It is valid only for sub-atomic particles which are so tiny and travel so fast that they approach the speed of light. It has nothing whatever to do with the vibrations of atoms in molecules, or of molecules in crystals or in solution.

I have gone into these ideas at some length because if scientific concepts are to be used to rationalize the mode of action of homeopathic drugs, they must provide scientific explanations. It is not enough to use terms like crystal field theory or wave-particle duality without explaining precisely what relevance these ideas have to homeopathic drug action. To use these theories out of context encourages scientists to reject the whole of homeopathic practice as unsound, whereas it is only the theory of the practice which may be scientifically untenable. The therapeutic procedures do have a reasonable degree of success.

24

ACUPUNCTURE

Physicians have been aware for centuries that disease in an organ of the body can cause pain in a completely different part of the anatomy – what they call 'referred pain'. Some common examples are the pains felt in the left arm from a heart condition, or in the chest from indigestion ('heartburn'), or in the back and lower abdomen from menstrual changes in the ovaries and uterus ('period pains').

The working principle of acupuncture therapy is similar: that there are sensitive points on the surface of the body which are connected through the nervous system to remote organs. When the organ is diseased, probing of these tender points with metal needles produces relief.

The Chinese, who originated acupuncture many thousands of years ago, explain the effectiveness of the technique in terms of Yin and Yang, negative and positive states of the body. Modern theory has it that acupuncture points correspond to positions where bundles of nerves are closest to the skin. Stimulation of these points by rotation of the stainless steel acupuncture needles generates nerve impulses to relieve pain.

The relief of pain (*analgesia*) and inducing a state of numbness to all sensation (*anaesthesia*) are the two main uses of acupuncture.

Acupuncturists sometimes enhance the effect of their technique by heating the needles or passing a small electric current through them. The corresponding electrical stimulation of the skin alone is said by some to relieve pain just as effectively as acupuncture. The process of burning mugwort (*Artemisia vulgaris*) to heat the ends of acupuncture needles is known as *moxibustion*.

Recent research has shown that during the stress of injury the body produces pain-killing chemicals which have a similar effect to the artificial pain-killing drug *morphine*. These compounds are chemically quite different from morphine; they are made up of strings of amino acids and are called *polypeptides*. However, since they behave like internal or endogenous morphine, they were called *endorphines*. Endorphines may contribute to long-term pain relief, but some researchers feel that they are unlikely to account for the instant relief that acupuncture can produce, since it takes several minutes for endorphine concentration to build up in tissues.

For an explanation of instant relief we may have to look to the mechanisms of nerve impulse transmissions. Messages are believed to travel by the release of chemicals (like *acetylcholine*) from the end of one nerve across the gaps between nerves (*synapses*) to be picked up by the sensors (*dendrites*) of the next nerve in the chain. All of this takes place instantly when we touch a hot surface, for example. Within a second or so, messages are flashed from the fingertips to the brain and back to the arm muscles for action. Acupuncture may involve a similar instant message transmission system with other pain-killing chemicals as yet undiscovered. We now know, for example, that rubbing the skin after we've received a blow does produce physiological healing effects at that site.

As well as relieving pain, acupuncture has been used for treating disorders as physically different as asthma and arthritis. It is claimed that it not only relieves the distressing symptoms but also produces some degree of remission of the disease.

A variation of acupuncture is to use fingertip pressure on the sensitive points instead of injecting needles. This technique is known as *acupressure* or *shiatsu*. The pressure points are called *tsubo*.

One possible criticism of acupuncture is that it may be used to mask pain from a diseased organ which requires treatment. Pain is the body's way of telling the owner that something is wrong. If the symptoms are cured without treatment of the cause, the patient can be worse off in the long term. The same argument could be used, however, against the treatment of symptoms by conventional drug therapy. Overall, acupuncture is one of the more successful alternative therapies and it is now gaining ground as one of the techniques used by orthodox physicians.

25

NEGATIVE ION THERAPY

Atoms and molecules of all the substances around us tend to be electrically neutral unless they are subjected to an electromagnetic field or they are themselves bombarded with charged particles. Then, particles of electricity (*electrons*) are often torn off the outer parts of the atoms. When this happens, the atoms or molecules become positively or negatively charged: positively charged if they lose a particle of electricity, negatively charged if they gain one. We say that the atoms or molecules have formed *ions*.

The effects of positive and negative ions on the human body, on animals, and on the growth of plants have been studied extensively for at least two decades in the West, and for sixty years or more in the USSR.

Positive ions have been found to produce negative or harmful effects on the body – lassitude, depression, headaches, anxiety, lack of concentration, susceptibility to respiratory tract infections – with subjects who are particularly sensitive. Those who are healthy and robust often describe feelings of euphoria and show hyperactivity from positive ions in the short term, but even they succumb to their debilitating effect in due course, though this may take weeks or months.

Negative ions, on the other hand, have been found, through a number of biological experiments and clinical trials around the world, to exert a positive or beneficial effect on the body.

Perhaps the most striking clinical results achieved by negative ion therapy are in the healing of wounds and burns, and for the treatment of respiratory diseases such as hay fever, catarrh and asthma. Many people report at least some relief from these problems and sometimes considerable benefit from negative ion therapy.

Negative ions also reduce blood pressure and pulse rate, produce a sense of well-being, and increase resistance to respiratory tract infection. They exert a generally calming effect, apparently by increasing the so-called alpha rhythms in the brain. By improving co-ordination between these alpha rhythms in different regions of the brain they increase concentration.

It seems that we react to stress in two different ways. When we are confronted with obvious danger, the 'fight-or-flight' mechanism triggers the release of two hormones from the central part (*medulla*) of our adrenal glands – *adrenaline* and *noradrenaline* (also called epinephrine and norepinephrine). Adrenaline and its close chemical partner, noradrenaline, increase heart rate and blood pressure but produce relaxation of the bronchial muscles and those of the gut – hence their use in injections for asthmatics. These chemicals are responsible for putting us on the alert if we have to take an examination or a driving test or make an important speech. A certain amount of this sort of stress is beneficial for us.

But there is another kind of stress. This is the subconscious emotional stress we experience when we have trauma in our lives, such as divorce, deaths of relatives, or losing a job. This releases another compound called *serotonin (5-hydroxytryptamine)* or 5HT. This also produces an elevation of heart rate and blood pressure (like adrenaline) but a contraction of the bronchial muscles and muscles of the gut, where it is largely concentrated in the body. Hence emotional stress tends to provoke wheeziness in asthmatics, and a tightening of the muscles in the gut in everyone.

This diversion into the workings of the nervous system is to explain the actions of positive and negative ions, as far as they are understood. Positive ions generate serotonin; negative ions promote conversion of serotonin into its complicated-sounding chemical end-product, 5HIAA (*5-hydroxyindoleacetic acid*).

Negative ion generators are now used in many offices to 'purify' the air and reduce the incidence of fatigue and headaches.

Unfortunately, many of our modern environments seem to promote a positive ion surplus and negative ion depletion. 'Stale' air in crowded offices and in large cities is not only poor in oxygen but also deficient in negative ions. Air-conditioning produces positive ions in the circulating air, the negative particles of electricity, ripped off the atoms by friction with the current of air, staying in the metal ducts.

Synthetic fabrics become positively charged by friction, the smaller negative particles escaping into the air. Our clothes then keep us immersed in a bath of positive ions which penetrate our bodies through the skin.

Negative ions are more concentrated in open areas, fields in the countryside, by the seashore, or in mountain areas – hence at least part of the health-giving properties of these environments, though the clean air and aesthetic qualities of such surroundings obviously make a contribution also.

Negative ions are generated by spraying water, as in waterfalls and sea spray, and perhaps even in domestic showers. Water ionizes into a positive part (*proton*) and a negative part (*hydroxyl*). The positive part stays with the uncharged water molecules (to form *hydroxonium ions*), while the smaller negative parts are more mobile. At least, that's the theory.

This is the rationale which is used to explain why humidifiers often bring relief to asthmatics, despite *increasing* the moisture in the air. The larger positive water droplets move downwards to the ground, while the negative ions circulate in the air to be inhaled. This benefit offsets what would be expected as a detrimental effect from increasing the air humidity. Asthmatics are generally more comfortable in dry air.

This, then, is the current thinking behind the mechanism of negative ion therapy. However it works (and many scientists and doctors are still sceptical), it has undoubtedly brought relief to numerous sufferers of headache, tension, insomnia, and nervous disorders; of asthma, rhinitis, and respiratory problems; and those who have suffered major burns.

For the healthy, negative ions promote mental alertness in the daytime but subsequent sound sleep at night, and are supposed also to improve libido or sex drive.

Part 4

REFERENCE SECTION

26

VITAMINS IN DETAIL

VITAMIN A

The term 'vitamin A' usually means vitamin A alcohol or *retinol*. (All chemicals belonging to the family of alcohols have names ending in -ol.) There is also a vitamin A aldehyde, *retinal* (-al, the aldehyde ending), and a vitamin A acid, *retinoic acid*, giving three compounds which are closely related chemically and which all have biological activity. We shall meet a comparable chemical family when pyridoxine (vitamin B6) is discussed (see page 154).

Metabolism: vitamin A is essential for healthy vision. It maintains the pliancy of the *cornea*, the hard transparent front surface of the eye. At the back of the eye there is a light-sensitive layer called the retina, which contains two types of light-detecting cells: rods and cones. Rods respond to low-intensity light; cones are triggered by bright light and distinguish between the light of different colours. In order to do this, these detectors contain a light-sensitive pigment, like the emulsion which coats a photographic film. (The rod pigment is *rhodopsin*, that in the cones is *iodopsin*; and the general name for either is *visual purple*.) Our bodies make this pigment from vitamin A, and they can produce vitamin A from a compound called *carotene* by simply chopping the latter molecule in half (and adding hydrogen).

Daily requirement: the US RDA value of vitamin A in adults is 3,300 International Units (IU), or 1,000 Retinol Equivalents, or 1 mg retinol. These are the three different sets of units which are used to express quantities of this vitamin. This amount corresponds to an intake of 6 mg of beta-carotene daily. (Only about one-third of the beta-carotene that we eat is absorbed, and only one-half of that is converted into vitamin A. So we need to eat six times as much beta-carotene in order to get our daily intake of vitamin A.) The UK RDA value is 2,500 International Units, or 750 mcg. The RDA value for infants under a year old is 450 mcg, increasing to 750 to 1,000 mcg at puberty. Women, with a lower average body weight than men, may need slightly less, except when they are pregnant or nursing, in which case the recommended intake is 1.2 mg (or 1,200 mcg) daily.

Food sources: the best food sources of vitamin A are whole milk, full-fat dairy produce, fish-liver oils, and eggs (the yolk), with somewhat less in liver and kidneys. Carotene comes from carrots and other red or yellow fruit and vegetables: tomatoes, sweet potatoes and apricots (oranges, although yellow, contain no carotene; they owe their yellow colour to another pigment called xanthophyll). One large, fresh, raw carrot may provide up to 10,000 IU vitamin A; one fresh, raw tomato up to 1,000 IU, in both cases as carotene, but the amount is highly variable (see Chapter 7).

Symptoms of deficiency or excess: lack of vitamin A causes a drying of the cornea (*xerophthalmia*) and difficulty with vision in dim light. Eventually, a deficiency will produce drying and hardening of the skin (*keratosis*) and lank hair.

An excess of vitamin A produces inflammation of the liver, where most of the vitamin is stored; pain in the joints; headache and nausea from increased fluid pressure in the central nervous system (brain and spinal chord); and yellow pigmentation of the skin.

Carrot or mixed vegetable juices are excellent nutrients, but under no circumstances should you drink large quantities of them daily. As with most things, the practical guideline is moderation, even with nutrients. You should limit your consumption of vegetable juice to about 250 ml (½ pint) per day. Doses of 50,000 IU daily can produce some of the symptoms of toxicity within a month or so in susceptible individuals.

VITAMIN B COMPLEX

Vitamin B is the most complicated of the vitamins because it consists of a mixture of many different compounds. It was the first vitamin to be characterized at the turn of the century when a Dutch physician, Christiaan Eijkman, found that beriberi could be prevented by a diet of whole-grain rice but not with polished rice. Eijkman was awarded the Nobel Prize in Physiology for his work in 1929, jointly with an English biochemist, Sir Frederick Hopkins, who did outstanding work on vitamins as well as in many other fields of medicine.

Thiamin or Vitamin B1

Metabolism: thiamin is found in the body in its diphosphate or pyrophosphate form, the phosphate groups being added as the thiamin passes through the small intestine. Half of this is in our muscles, the other half divided between our principal organs – the heart, brain, liver and kidneys.

Thiamin diphosphate is a coenzyme in many reactions involved in carbohydrate metabolism and thus helps to maintain muscle tone, appetite and general vigour. We cannot use carbohydrates for energy without it. Its other principal function is to maintain a healthy nervous system.

Daily requirement: for the adult male the RDA value is 1.7 mg (US) or 1.4 mg (UK), with proportionately lower amounts for women and children, who have a lower body weight.

Food sources: thiamin is found in whole-grain cereals and yeast, with smaller amounts in nuts and legumes.

Symptoms of deficiency or excess: a deficiency of this vitamin produces beriberi, with inflammation of the nerves (*polyneuritis*), wasting of the tissues (*emaciation*), accumulation of fluid, especially in the limbs (*oedema*), loss of appetite (*anorexia*), and enlargement and impaired function of the heart.

There are no known toxic effects of excess of thiamin, though an intake of more than 1 g daily may produce diuresis (excessive urination).

Riboflavin or Vitamin B2

Metabolism: this is needed to keep our skin and other body tissues in a healthy condition. It forms part of two coenzymes which act as charge carriers in the oxidation of fats, carbohydrates and proteins (*see* metabolism of niacin, below).

Daily requirement: the RDA value is 1.5 to 1.8 mg for adults, with amounts for children in proportion to their body weight.

Food sources: best sources of the vitamin are whole-grain cereals, yeast, dairy produce, eggs and offal (kidney, liver and heart), with less in green, leafy vegetables, legumes and meat. The riboflavin in milk may be deactivated by the action of light when it is stored in clear glass bottles.

Symptoms of deficiency or excess: deficiency of riboflavin produces skin lesions which may appear first of all in the scalp (*seborrhoea*), lips (*chellosis*), eyes (*conjunctivitis*) and, in men, the scrotum (*scrotal dermatitis*).

No symptoms of excess have been described.

Niacin

Sometimes designated as vitamin B3 (or B5). The chemical name for niacin is nicotinic acid, which gets its name from nicotine, from which it is easily prepared by oxidation. The body does *not* turn nicotine into niacin or vice versa.

There is also a chemically modified version of niacin called niacinamide (or, chemically, *nicotinamide*). Both show vitamin activity in our bodies.

Metabolism: the principal physiological role of niacin is to form part of two vital coenzymes involved in many of the body's reactions but particularly those concerned with tissue maintenance. They work in a complementary fashion to the coenzymes produced from riboflavin.

The body can manufacture 1 mg of niacin from approximately 60 mg of the amino acid *tryptophan*.

Daily requirement: the RDA value is 15 to 20 mg for adults, 5 mg for infants under one year old, with amounts for children in proportion to their body weight. Pregnant and lactating women should ensure they get at least 18 to 21 mg daily, the respective UK RDA values.

Food sources: as with the other B vitamins mentioned so far, niacin is found in whole-grain cereals, yeast, offal (kidney and liver), muscle meat, poultry and legumes (including peanuts). Milk is low in niacin but high in tryptophan, from which the body can make niacin.

Symptoms of deficiency or excess: deficiency in niacin produces *pellagra*, in which there is a deterioration of the tissue linings of the body (*epithelial tissues*): the skin (producing dermatitis), the gastrointestinal tract (giving rise to anorexia and diarrhoea), and the linings of the central nervous system (leading to insomnia, irritability, depression and eventually dementia).

Apart from some reversible pigmentation of the skin, an excess of niacin produces no known symptoms of toxicity in healthy individuals. People with diabetes or peptic ulcers may be more susceptible, however, and should never take niacin supplement tablets without medical supervision.

Pantothenic acid

Also called vitamin B5 (or B3 – *see* niacin, opposite).

Metabolism: pantothenic acid is found in all living tissues, with concentrations in the brain, liver and kidneys. It is used in the body mainly for conversion to a coenzyme which is involved in many of the body's chemical reactions, particularly those concerned with lipid and carbohydrate metabolism and the release of energy.

Pantothenic acid is also a part of another coenzyme which is concerned with fatty-acid metabolism.

Although it restores colour to grey hair in rats, pantothenic acid has never been shown to have a comparable effect in man.

Daily requirement: no RDA level has been established because so many foods contain pantothenic acid and it is distributed so widely in the body. Daily intake levels of 5 and 10 mg for children and adults respectively have been tentatively suggested as desirable.

Food sources: pantothenic acid is found in most plant and animal tissues, as its name suggests (Greek: *pantothene* – from everywhere). Richest sources, as for some of the other B vitamins, are whole-grain cereals, yeast, eggs (the yolk), offal (liver, kidney and brain), fresh vegetables, milk and dairy produce.

Symptoms of deficiency or excess: deficiency, rarely encountered in normal circumstances, causes irritability, restlessness, insomnia, fatigue, poor co-ordination, and gastrointestinal problems.

It has also been shown recently that deficiency of either pantothenic acid or pyridoxine results in a failure to manufacture antibodies against infection, the failure being most marked if both vitamins are lacking. It is therefore recommended by naturopaths in doses of up to 100 mg daily for those susceptible to respiratory tract infections or allergic reactions, though it has not been established, either theoretically or experimentally, that this measure does produce real improvements. (Note: even if a deficiency state of a nutrient is defined, an excess of that nutrient may not produce relief of similar symptoms in other individuals.)

Tablet supplements of pantothenic acid are usually in the form of the calcium salt. Of every 100 mg of calcium pantothenate, roughly 90 mg is pantothenate and 10 mg calcium.

No symptoms of excess of pantothenic acid have been recorded.

Pyridoxine or Vitamin B6

Pyridoxine, strictly speaking, is an alcohol and is therefore also known as *pyridoxol*. There are two other compounds with vitamin B6 activity – the aldehyde *pyridoxal* and an amino derivative, *pyridoxamine* (with an amine group, like amino acids). The word 'pyridoxine' is sometimes used to mean just the alcohol and sometimes any or all of the three compounds with vitamin B6 activity. It is probably least confusing to adopt the latter convention.

Metabolism: present in most of the body's tissues, vitamin B6 again forms coenzymes, like other B vitamins. It occurs as the phosphate in coenzymes concerned with protein metabolism.

Daily requirement: the US RDA value is 2 mg for adults and 0.5 to 1 mg for children between one and ten years old.

Food sources: pyridoxol is found mainly in fruit and vegetables, and pyridoxal and pyridoxamine occur primarily in animal produce.

Vitamin B6 is found in all such tissues: meats, offal, dairy produce, eggs, nuts, fresh fruit and vegetables, fish, etc. There are no special recommended sources. The vitamin is easily destroyed in food processing, however.

Symptoms of deficiency or excess: as for pantothenic acid, a deficiency of pyridoxine results in a failure to manufacture antibodies against infection.

Since this vitamin in the form of its coenzymes is involved primarily in protein metabolism, the deficiency also leads to deterioration of the body's tissues. The effects are seen first in disorders of the skin and nerves, as with other B vitamins, producing nervousness, irritability, fatigue, insomnia, skin lesions and ultimately convulsions and anaemia. With B1, B3 and B5, it is a common constituent of naturopathic remedies for nervous tension and insomnia (*see* note in paragraph on deficiency state of pantothenic acid, above).

Many women who suffer from pre-menstrual tension have been helped by daily tablet supplements of 40 to 80 mg of pyridoxine, but the mechanism of action has not been established.

An excess of vitamin B6 may also produce restlessness and insomnia. To reach this state most people would probably require something in excess of 100 mg daily, but again, susceptible individuals may experience side effects with much lower doses.

Cyanocobalamin or Vitamin B12

As its name suggests, this compound contains cobalt: each molecule contains one atom of cobalt situated at the centre of a ring structure (*porphyrin*), much like the iron in haem. It also contains a cyanide group which, in this environment, is quite harmless. It's rather like the difference between chlorine gas, which is a deadly poison, and the harmless chloride ions we have in our bodies. The cyanide ion is highly poisonous, but vitamin B12 contains a cyanide radical. We also need the mineral phosphorus to make up the B12 molecule.

There are also other compounds with B12 activity (*hydroxocobalamin* and *nitritocobalamin*).

Metabolism: in order to absorb vitamin B12 into the intestinal wall we must secrete a special protein from the stomach. This complex is then linked up to calcium so that it can pass into the intestinal cells. Here the B12 is released and transferred to a cell protein to carry it through the cell wall into the blood stream. This protein in turn hands the B12 on to a blood serum protein (*transcobalamin*) for transport to the blood-forming tissues. It's rather like a biological relay race with vitamin B12 as the baton.

The presence of vitamin B12 is necessary to enable us to make red blood cells (*erythrocytes*) in the hollow tubes in the centres of our bones (a process called *haemopoiesis*). These spaces are filled with red and yellow bone marrow and it is here that the red and some of our white blood cells are made (the rest of the white blood cells are made in the lymph glands).

Vitamin B12 is also used in the metabolism of nucleic acids (in the centres or nuclei of our cells) and for the normal functioning of the vitamin folacin (see below). Both these operations are also involved in the healthy blood cell formation just described.

Daily requirement: the US RDA value is only 3 mcg for an adult.

Food sources: animal tissue is the main source of vitamin B12. Cereals, fruit and vegetables contain almost none. There is some in milk and dairy produce, eggs and brewer's yeast, which provide alternative sources for vegetarians. Vegans are recommended to take a tablet supplement.

No mechanism for manufacture of B12 in the body has yet been established, although as the red blood cell count of people fed on cobalt salts does increase, some mechanism almost certainly exists. Cobalt salts are widespread in nature in green, leafy vegetables (see page 178).

Symptoms of deficiency or excess: vitamin B12 deficiency states are well known. A lack of this vitamin produces *anaemia*, if the diet or absorption of the vitamin are inadequate, and *pernicious anaemia*, usually in the elderly, if there is an inherited genetic defect. Fatigue, depression, restlessness, irritability and stiffness of the limbs are typical symptoms of anaemia.

No symptoms of vitamin B12 excess have been defined.

Folacin

This is also known as folic acid. Once the acidic hydrogens have been split off, the active part of the molecule is called *folate*.

Metabolism: folacin functions as a coenzyme which helps to build up organic molecules. For example, it converts the amino acids *glycine* and *homocysteine* into *serine* and *methionine* respectively.

Folacin coenzymes also participate in the body's synthesis of *choline* (see page 158); in the amino acid conversion of *phenylalanine* into *tyrosine*; in the synthesis of components of nucleic acids; and in the manufacture of red blood cells (*erythrocytes*) in the bone marrow.

Daily requirement: the US RDA value for folacin is 400 mcg for a 64 kg (10 stone) adult, with amounts for children in proportion to their body weight.

Food sources: folacin is widely distributed in green, leafy vegetables – hence its name (Latin: *folium* – leaf). It is also found in raw fruit. It occurs as free folacin, which is readily absorbed by the intestine; or bound to further glutamic acid molecules, which have to be processed by our digestion before we can use the folate.

Symptoms of deficiency or excess: deficiency of folacin causes anaemia, gastrointestinal disturbances and diarrhoea; these may be brought about by either inadequate dietary supply or poor absorption. Though the evidence cannot yet be regarded as conclusive, there are strong indications from an increasing body of data that neural defects of the newborn, including spina bifida, may be the result of folacin deficiencies in the mother during pregnancy.

An excess of folacin is not known to be toxic, but as it works with cyanocobalamin in the production of red blood corpuscles, high doses – several milligrams each day – may mask the symptoms of anaemia in the early stages, and the disease can be more dangerous if treatment is delayed.

PABA or para-aminobenzoic acid

This is a part, structurally, of folacin. Although the food sources in which it is most abundant (whole cereal grains) are different from those in which folacin occurs, PABA's main physiological function seems to be to act as the starting point (*precursor*) for the body's manufacture of folacin.

Biotin

This is part of the vitamin B complex but is also known as vitamin H, though this term is not often used nowadays.

Metabolism: biotin is used in the metabolism of proteins, carbohydrates and lipids, and to make the larger fatty-acid molecules.

The absorption of biotin from the intestine is prevented by raw egg white, which contains a protein-carbohydrate complex called *avidin*. Fortunately, this is easily denatured by cooking, which then allows biotin absorption to proceed normally.

Bacteria in our intestines make up to six times as much biotin as we need.

Daily requirement: no specified requirement has been established since we can apparently synthesize as much as we require in the gut.

Food sources: apart from what our bodies manufacture, biotin is widely distributed in plant and animal foods: offal (kidney and liver), poultry, eggs (the yolk), milk, and fresh vegetables. Meat and cereals contain little biotin.

Symptoms of deficiency or excess: none has been defined. As we make our own biotin in the gut and it is available from so many foods, deficiency is not likely to be a problem. Excess biotin is excreted in both urine and faeces.

Choline

This is included by some as part of the vitamin B complex, but others regard it as a lipid.

Metabolism: choline, joined together with glycerol and phosphate, forms a phospholipid, *lecithin*. As such, it is an integral part of the membrane of the cells of our bodies. Lecithin acts to reduce the level of fatty acids and cholesterol circulating in the blood stream.

Choline is the starting material (*precursor*) for *acetylcholine*, which we need for sending messages along our nerves.

Choline also functions to make molecules in our bodies bigger by adding on carbon atoms.

Daily requirement: none has been established, but on a normal diet we consume about 1 g daily.

Food sources: these are widely distributed, but the richest sources of choline are offal (brain, liver and kidneys), muscle meat, dairy produce, eggs and whole-grain cereals.

Symptoms of deficiency or excess: none has been defined.

Inositol

Metabolism: inositol seems to work in the body in some way with biotin and choline, but its precise function is not known. It is certainly involved in lipid metabolism as one of the alternative alcohols to glycerol in phospholipids. Inositol is concentrated in the nerves and semen.

Daily requirement: no value has been established as inositol occurs widely in food and we appear to be able to synthesize it in the intestines.

Food sources: most abundant sources are offal (kidneys and liver) and whole-grain cereals, with smaller amounts in fruit and vegetables. In cereals, inositol is found joined together chemically with phosphoric acid (*phosphoinositol*) in the form of its calcium/magnesium salt (known as *phytin*).

Symptoms of deficiency or excess: none has been defined.

ASCORBIC ACID OR VITAMIN C

This is the only vitamin which is a single compound, and it was the first to be isolated as a chemically pure substance. This was achieved in 1928 by the Hungarian biochemist Albert Szent-Györgyi, who was awarded the Nobel Prize in physiology in 1937 for his work. Now over 90, he is still scientifically active.

Like phenol, ascorbic acid is a weak acid and forms a monosodium salt, sodium ascorbate, which is one of the forms available as tablet supplements of the vitamin. The active portion of vitamin C is the *ascorbate* ion, which is a strong reducing agent, that is, it readily donates unit negative charges (*electrons*) or hydrogen atoms to other molecules. These negative charges are needed in many essential biochemical reactions.

Metabolism: vitamin C is rapidly absorbed from the intestine into the blood stream and distributed to most tissues of the body, particularly those with high metabolic activity, like the liver and the brain. It is used in protein and lipid metabolism, especially in the formation of connective tissue protein, *collagen*, found in skin, bone and cartilage. Ascorbate participates in the conversion of cholesterol into bile acids in the liver. It thus contributes to a lowering of blood cholesterol and to efficient digestion of lipids.

With ATP (*adenosine triphosphate*) and magnesium, ascorbate acts as cofactor to an enzyme which switches off the body's mechanism for burning fatty acids as food, once our energy requirements have been met.

Absorption of iron into soluble tissue iron-protein (*ferritin*) and the activity of folacin in red blood cell formation (*see* vitamin B, page 157) both require ascorbate.

The healthy adult body contains about 1.5 g of ascorbate. Excesses are excreted by the kidneys into the urine.

Daily requirement: this is a highly contentious issue which is discussed at length here in the section on symptoms of deficiency or excess. The RDA value is 60 mg (US) or 30 mg (UK), except for pregnant or lactating women, for which the UK RDA value is 60 mg. Experimental evidence exists to show that people who take drugs daily, including oral contraceptives, tobacco or alcohol, benefit from two or three times this amount.

Only primates and guinea pigs need to take vitamin C in their diet. Other animals and plants can make it for themselves from a single-unit sugar to which ascorbic acid is closely related chemically.

Food sources: fresh fruit and vegetables are the principal sources of this vitamin. Dairy produce, meat and cereals contain little. The foods richest in vitamin C are blackcurrants, rosehips and citrus fruits; and green, leafy vegetables like Brussels sprouts and cabbage.

Vitamin C is quite unstable to both heat and light. Its content in food will be diminished by cooking or prolonged storage, particularly in the light. It is also readily soluble in water. The presence of copper or iron, which are good absorbers of negative charges, hastens the destruction of ascorbate.

Symptoms of deficiency or excess: it has been known since the mid-eighteenth century that fresh fruit prevents the disease of the connective tissues called scurvy. James Lind, the English physician, recommended fresh oranges or lemons be included in the diet of sailors on long voyages. Scurvy is characterized by general weakness of the limbs, bleeding and deterioration of the tissues of the gums, spotty appearance of the skin as haemorrhages develop around the hair follicles, and the failure of wounds to heal. Vitamin C is therefore the anti-scorbutic factor (hence, ascorbic acid). 30 mg of ascorbate daily will certainly prevent scurvy, but this may not be nearly enough for general health.

Increased doses of vitamin C above the RDA value can provide added protection against ill health – that much is now established beyond reasonable doubt. The two contentious issues which remain are:

1   How much extra vitamin C do we need? Is 100 mg or so enough, or do we need the megadoses recommended by Linus Pauling and others? This is a difficult question to answer because so little is known about the absorption and protection of vitamin C in the body.
2   What precisely does vitamin C do? Does it give added protection against the effects of stress and respiratory tract infection, and is it also beneficial in preventing atherosclerosis and cancer in the long term?

These questions cannot be answered with certainty at present. Some studies have found direct or circumstantial statistical evidence that vitamin C does produce these benefits; other studies have proved negative. There are many factors that may contribute to this discrepancy.

The various studies have involved different doses of the vitamin, administered in different ways (orally or by injection), for various periods of time, in different forms (using ascorbic acid, sodium ascorbate or calcium ascorbate), and given at different times of the day (in a single or multiple dose, on a full or empty stomach). Furthermore, the vitamin potency is often not assessed immediately prior to use; and vitamin C, as mentioned above, deteriorates rapidly in solution and in the presence of light, copper or iron. Finally, some studies have not involved enough subjects for statistical data to be reliably interpreted, taking into account the biochemical individuality which has been stressed throughout this book.

There are similar variations in the reporting of adverse effects of excess vitamin C. Ascorbic acid is a weak acid, weaker than those found in oranges and lemons (*citrus acid*), grapes (*tartaric acid*), or sour milk (*lactic acid*). It is, however, stronger than the acid in vinegar (*acetic acid*), and it may be this acidity which produces the gastric irritation reported by some people who take high doses. On the other hand, there are also cases where gastritis has actually been treated with high doses of vitamin C. Again, it is a question of differences between the reactions of various individuals.

Some researchers claim that megadoses of vitamin C cause kidney stones for those who have a predisposition to this problem. Kidney stones come in two varieties. People with acidic urine may form stones of calcium oxalate, uric acid or cystine. If the tendency to formation of these stones already exists, a high intake of vitamin C (of the order of 1 g daily) may aggravate the problem. People tending to formation of stones of calcium or magnesium carbonates or phosphates have alkaline urine, and the condition is more likely to be alleviated than worsened by vitamin C.

In view of the controversy about the effects of megadoses, the most reasonable compromise is to take 200 to 600 mg of vitamin C daily by tablet supplement, on an empty stomach and preferably accompanied by an acid drink of fruit juice. This dosage is unlikely to cause kidney stone formation unless you know you have this problem already; in which case you should stick to the 30 to 60 mg RDA value. You should also decrease your dose back to this level if you experience nausea, indigestion or diarrhoea which you can attribute to high ascorbic acid intake and not to fruit juice or other components of your diet. For other people, this increased daily intake is likely to be beneficial, though how beneficial is at this stage a matter of individual opinion.

CALCIFEROL OR VITAMIN D

There are two main compounds that have vitamin D activity. We can either get these directly in our food or make them in the body by a series of chemical reactions from two other very similar compounds. The two starting materials are known as *provitamins D*. One provitamin D is called *ergosterol* and this is changed into *ergocalciferol* (vitamin D2); the other is *7-dehydrocholesterol* (cholesterol with two hydrogen atoms missing) and this is converted into *cholecalciferol* (vitamin D3). (There is no vitamin D1 any longer – this was found to be a mixture.) As their names suggest, both provitamins D are closely related to the steroids.

Metabolism: our bodies can carry out these conversions of provitamins D into the active vitamin with the help of ultraviolet light from the sun. One benefit of a limited amount of sunlight, therefore, is that it enables us to make vitamin D, which is absorbed directly through the skin into the blood stream.

Vitamin D in the diet is absorbed by the intestine and fed into the lymph system, along with other lipids.

Vitamin D is activated by chemical changes carried out successively in the liver and kidneys to form a still more potent vitamin which is responsible for increased absorption of calcium and phosphorus from the intestine, and deposition of the inorganic material of our bones.

Daily requirement: the US RDA value for vitamin D is 400 IU or 10 mcg daily for infants, children or adults, and the UK RDA value is 10 mcg for children and pregnant or lactating women, and 100 IU or 2.5 mcg for adult men and women.

Food sources: the plant provitamin D is ergosterol; the one in animals is 7-dehydrocholesterol. Milk and dairy produce, eggs (the yolk), fish-liver oils and animal livers are the best sources of vitamin D. Milk is often fortified with up to 10 mcg of vitamin D per 1.1 l (2 pints). A 30 g (1 oz) serving of breakfast cereal will give you about 1 mcg. We also get a significant amount from irradiation of the skin by sunlight, but precisely how much depends on the intensity of exposure, which in turn is dependent on many factors: altitude, season, time of day, cloud cover, air pollution, etc.

Symptoms of deficiency or excess: deficiency states of vitamin D are well known. Without vitamin D, children's bones are soft and bend under their body weight, leading to the development of bow legs and knock knees, and enlargement of the joints, a condition known as rickets.

Slight excesses of vitamin D are excreted through the faeces. A high excess, certainly above 50 mcg daily, may lead to *hypercalcaemia*, where calcium is deposited in the kidneys and then the other organs, as a result of which they can be irreversibly damaged.

Unless you work habitually on night shift or are a vegan, so that the normal sources of vitamin D are not available to you, you don't require a tablet supplement. Indeed, anything more than minimal supplementation may actually do you harm.

TOCOPHEROL OR VITAMIN E

There are eight closely related compounds with vitamin E activity: alpha-, beta-, gamma- and delta-tocopherol, and alpha-, beta-, gamma-

and delta-tocotrienol. The most potent is alpha-tocopherol; beta-, gamma- and delta-tocopherol have only 40 per cent, 8 per cent and 1 per cent respectively of the biological activity of the alpha form.

Metabolism: little is known yet of the metabolism of vitamin E. It is an anti-sterility factor (Greek: *tokos* – offspring; *pherein* – to bear). It is necessary for the vitality of sex cells, but does nothing apparently for sexual vigour. It is absorbed directly from the intestine into the lymph system with the other fat-soluble vitamins.

Its main role in the body seems to be to act as an antioxidant – preventing deterioration of polyunsaturated compounds like vitamin A or fatty acids. Such oxidation is carried out by *radicals*, groups of atoms which seek out negative charges (*electrons*) that they can take away from other molecules. Unsaturated compounds are always rich in loosely bound negative charges. Tocopherols have been used in this way for many years in the processing of food to prevent fats becoming rancid.

Vitamin E also works in combination with or as an alternative to selenium in the antioxidant role, and seems to protect vitamin C, which is both unsaturated and unstable.

Vitamin E is stored in most organs of the body and body fat. The healthy plasma concentration of vitamin E should be about 1 mg/100 ml, of which more than 80 per cent is alpha-tocopherol.

Daily requirement: the US RDA value of vitamin E for adult males is 15 IU and for adult females 12 IU, approximately equivalent to 12 and 10 mg of alpha-tocopherol respectively.

Food sources: wheatgerm oil is by far the richest natural source of vitamin E. In a normal diet we get the vitamin from whole-grain cereals, nuts, legumes and leafy, green vegetable and salad foods. Vitamin E, like the vitamin C it protects, is itself unstable and is easily destroyed by heating or ultraviolet light. Tablet supplements of vitamin E often contain additives to prolong the life of the vitamin.

Symptoms of deficiency or excess: a deficiency of vitamin E leads to sterility and muscular dystrophy (wasting) in animals. Whether a deficiency of the vitamin has the same effect on humans has not yet been established.

A slight excess of vitamin E (up to 100 mg daily) is certainly not toxic to humans. High doses *are* toxic in animals, and if health food devotees want to extrapolate the benefits of the vitamin in animals to imply comparable benefits in humans, then the toxicity of high doses of the vitamin in animals should not be ignored. In susceptible individuals even 50 mg daily may produce indigestion, diarrhoea and palpitations, the most common side effects from excess intake.

There is no convincing experimental evidence that the vitamin has any beneficial effect either in humans or animals on wound healing, sexual desire or in delaying the ageing process. The best that can be said for it is that it is almost certainly an essential nutrient (there may be dietary alternatives), which maintains the health of cells generally, and in this respect should help prolong all normal body functions and inhibit their deterioration with age or through disease.

VITAMIN F

Vitamin F is the old name for the essential fatty acids – linoleic, linolenic and arachidonic (see page 32).

VITAMIN H

This is the old name for biotin (see page 157).

VITAMIN K

Vitamin K consists of two groups of yellow-coloured substances denoted as vitamins K1 (also called *phylloquinone*) and K2; and there are several synthetic compounds which have vitamin K activity. Natural vitamin K has a long polyunsaturated chain of carbon (and hydrogen) atoms, just like the polyunsaturated fatty acids, and this makes them soluble in fats but insoluble in water; the chain also increases their vitamin K activity. There is experimental evidence to suggest that they may have a physiological role comparable to that of the unsaturated acids. Some of the synthetic compounds with vitamin K activity have the advantage of being soluble in water.

All vitamins K are chemical derivatives of naphthalene (familiar in its use as mothballs). They are stable to heat but unstable to light.

Metabolism: vitamin K is synthesized by bacteria in the gut and functions as a blood-clotting agent: it is an anti-haemorrhagic factor. Antibiotics like neomycin reduce this bacterial activity, lowering or stopping production of vitamin K in the intestine. Vitamin K requires the secretion of bile acids for its solution and absorption, which therefore occur much less efficiently in cases of liver or gall bladder disease.

Daily requirement: no daily intake level has been established, but the need is small and we appear to synthesize all we require under normal circumstances. We eat several milligrams of vitamin K in our food and we probably extract from this as much as we need to supplement what we synthesize.

Food sources: vitamin K, primarily as K1, is most abundant in green vegetables. Bacterial synthesis provides mainly (exclusively?) K2. Meat and dairy produce contain a little vitamin K, but cereals and fruits have almost none.

Symptoms of deficiency or excess: deficiencies are rarely met because of widespread food sources and synthesis of the vitamin in the body, but when encountered they are characterized by an increase in bleeding time – the time taken for blood from a fresh wound to clot.

There are no known symptoms of excess vitamin K intake, but tablet supplements should never be taken without medical supervision since they could promote thrombosis – the formation of blood clots in the arteries. It is particularly important that people on anticoagulant therapy should minimize their intake of foods rich in vitamin K.

BIOFLAVONOIDS OR VITAMIN P

Evidence collected over the past two or three decades suggests that these compounds are not vitamins at all. It was formerly thought that they increased the permeability of our blood vessels (hence P for permeability), allowing nutrients to pass from the tiny capillaries into our tissues. They occur naturally with vitamin C and may assist its metabolism in some way, but they don't appear to have any vitamin activity by themselves.

27

MINERALS IN DETAIL

SODIUM

Metabolism: sodium is used to maintain the fluid level in the body, and it is involved in the contraction of muscles and in nerve transmission.

If sodium is depleted, water moves into the cells and there is a drop in blood pressure. This causes the kidneys to release the enzyme *renin*, which in turn produces *aldosterone* from the adrenal gland. This makes the kidney conserve sodium and raises the blood pressure back to normal.

Daily requirement: because sodium is so widely distributed in foods, for the past few decades nutritionists and doctors have believed we may be getting too much in our diets. For this mineral, we are seeking generally to avoid rather than to obtain sodium in the diet unless there is a specific requirement for it.

Normal daily intake should be about 1.2 g of sodium or 3 g of common salt (sodium chloride). The healthy body has an efficient regulating system for sodium. It is lost through urine and sweating, so the daily requirement should be related to water intake, with 1 g of sodium per litre (1¾ pints) of water. Those who live in hot climates or who do heavy manual work will perspire more and will need to drink more. Even those who regularly play physically demanding sports like squash will during a game perspire much more than normal, losing perhaps as much as 2 l (3½ pints) per hour instead of 1 l (1¾ pints) per day.

Drinking more water to replace this lost fluid should always be accompanied by a corresponding amount of salt; but not at the same time, however. Salt water is an emetic: at the very least it is likely to produce nausea. The thing to do is to take one or two salt tablets (each usually containing 300 to 500 mg of salt) an hour or so before exertion. Sweating plus the extra water you drink during and after exertion will flush the excess through the system.

Food sources: foods which contain the most sodium, as salt, are bacon and ham, salted crackers and potato crisps, chips and tinned food. The last of these may also contain sodium as monosodium glutamate, which is added to enhance flavour. In addition, tinned meats have sodium nitrate or nitrite (E250 and E251) as a preservative to kill bacteria which might cause botulism.

Sodium bicarbonate, sodium aluminium sulphate and sodium pyrophosphate are common ingredients of baking powders. The sodium part remains intact in the cooking process so it will be present in most cakes and some biscuits. Sodium bicarbonate is also present in many antacids taken for indigestion, although there are some brands which are sodium-free.

Sodium citrate (E331) is an antioxidant used in processed cheeses. Sodium benzoate (E211) is widely used as a preservative in a whole range of food products – it is also highly suspect as a cause of food hypersensitivity, especially in children.

This is enough to give you an indication of how widespread sodium compounds are as food additives, quite apart from the natural sodium content of foods. Even fresh meat and fish contain more salt than fruit and vegetables, and sea fish more than fresh-water ones. Celery, carrots and spinach are the only common vegetables which are relatively high in salt content.

The average diet is likely to contain at least 3 g of sodium daily, more than double that which is normally required, and some people take much more than this.

Symptoms of deficiency or excess: sodium deficiency is only encountered in people who go through a period of vomiting and diarrhoea, or who are taking diuretics or adrenocortical hormones, like cortisol, for arthritis. Ephedrine, taken by asthmatics, may have a similar effect and, as noted above, profuse sweating may produce a short-term depletion.

Some people claim that small, concentrated doses (of 500 mg to 1 g) of salt daily help in the rapid healing of cold sores (herpes simplex lesions) or prevent their eruption. If this is so, this condition may represent a minor depletion state.

Sodium depletion (it rarely reaches the state of a deficiency) may be accompanied by fatigue and irritability. If the condition is such that it does deteriorate into a deficiency, as in heat stroke, unconsciousness may result.

Excess of sodium produces swelling of the joints (*oedema*) due to the accumulation of fluid.

A sodium-restricted diet is recommended for those who suffer from hypertension or congestive heart disease, kidney or liver malfunction, and also if toxaemia develops during pregnancy. In these cases, all preserved meats and tinned foods must be eliminated from the diet, and salt should not be added in food preparation. Mineral waters, which may be relatively high in sodium, should also be avoided. There are various herbs and spices which can be used instead of salt to give flavour to a low-sodium diet. Although sodium isn't believed to *cause* high blood pressure, it does seem to aggravate the condition. There are studies, however, which suggest that it isn't so much high sodium but low potassium (together with low phosphorus, calcium and vitamins A and C) which causes the problem. If this is proved to be the case, the condition could be improved, as the researchers suggest, by a diet rich in dairy produce! This argument has not yet been substantiated by other researchers.

As a general rule, you should aim to minimize your intake of salt even if you have no pathological condition, since you will get adequate amounts daily from whole, fresh food. Increase salt intake only if you lose it through sweating.

POTASSIUM

Metabolism: one use of potassium is to maintain the salt/water balance in tissues. It is the most abundant positive metal ion inside the cell (in *intracellular fluid*) and it operates in a complementary fashion with sodium, which is concentrated in the fluid outside the cell.

When muscles contract or when electrical or chemical impulses flow along nerve fibres, potassium diffuses out of the cells while sodium moves in. When the muscle or nerve fibres relax, the reverse chemical changes occur.

In order that the water-soluble potassium and sodium ions can pass through the organic lipid membrane wall of the cell they have to be wrapped up themselves in organic molecules called *ionophores*. These are ring-shaped organic molecules, rather like the haem of haemoglobin, with the metal ions in the middle. They replace the watery coat that metal ions have when they are in aqueous solution, like the blood. The first ionophore to be discovered was *valinomycin*, which likes to surround potassium ions; the ionophore *monensin* has an affinity for sodium, so between them they transport these two metal ions back and forth, into and out of the cells in our bodies.

Potassium activates the enzyme which begins the conversion of fructose into glucose, and it is also used in conjunction with other enzymes involved in the digestion of carbohydrates.

The human body contains about 2.6 g of potassium for every kilogram of weight. This means that a person weighing 64 kg (10 stone) will have 166 g of potassium in his body.

Daily requirement: we need about 3 g of potassium (just under 6 g of potassium chloride) each day. A balanced diet provides this without difficulty.

What matters most with potassium is not so much the absolute value of daily intake as the quantity in relation to sodium. The two must always be kept in balance by the body in a potassium/sodium ratio of about 2:1.

Only in cases of vomiting or diarrhoea, extensive burns, or with continued administration of drugs such as cortisol or diuretics is increased potassium intake recommended. In these conditions, it is better to get the potassium from food sources rather than tablets of potassium chloride; this compound is poorly absorbed and may have undesirable long-term effects.

Food sources: the best sources of potassium are milk, meat and fresh vegetables. 150 g (5¼ oz) of chicken provides 620 mg of potassium; 90 g (3 oz) warmed frozen peas, 120 mg; 1 medium (150 g/5¼ oz) potato, baked in its jacket, then peeled, gives another 780 mg – in total, half the daily requirement from a typical cooked dinner. Tinned salmon is also a good source, with a 90 g (3 oz) serving providing 300 mg.

There is 485 mg of potassium in 250 ml (½ pint) of milk. Full-fat cheese has 1 mg/g so a normal 90 g (3 oz) serving will supply 90 mg. Cottage cheese will supply little if the cream has been removed, since this is where most of the potassium comes from. (In some places cottage cheese can be bought as a plain or creamed variety.)

Amongst fruits, one avocado will provide between 1,000 and 2,000 mg of potassium. Bananas and apricots are the common fruits richest in potassium: one 100 g (3½ oz) banana gives 400 mg, while a 100 g (3½ oz) portion of apricots contains about 300 mg. Even a medium-sized apple (150 g/5¼ oz) will give 160 mg of potassium. Grapes and grapefruit are other rich sources.

Symptoms of deficiency or excess: as there are so many sources of potassium in the diet, deficiencies or excesses are rare.

Symptoms of potassium deficiency are lethargy and muscle weakness. An excess of potassium will only arise in cases of kidney malfunction, and the main effect is on the action of the heart.

Natural liquorice contains compounds that lower blood potassium (a condition known as *hypokalemia*), but only those who have a passion for large quantities of liquorice are likely to be affected. Liquorice should be avoided, however, by people with cardiovascular disease.

MAGNESIUM

Metabolism: adults have about 20 g of magnesium in their bodies. About half of this occurs as the carbonate alongside calcium in the bones. The remainder is in the soft tissues of the body, since magnesium plays a major role in activating a wide range of enzymes: for example, the enzyme which begins the breakdown of glucose to carbon dioxide and water to provide energy.

Magnesium participates in the reactions of other enzymes involved in carbohydrate digestion and energy transfer, as well as activating some protein-breaking enzymes.

Like calcium, magnesium is involved in nerve impulse transmission and muscle contraction/relaxation biochemistry, sometimes assisting calcium and sometimes opposing it.

In many systems of the body magnesium absorption increases if the intake of calcium is inadequate, but vitamin D is not involved in the absorption of magnesium, as it is in the absorption of calcium. Magnesium is essential for the uptake of vitamins, especially those of the B complex.

Plants also need magnesium in order to make chlorophyll, which has a structure very like the haem in our blood, except magnesium replaces the haem iron at the centre of the molecule. Plants use chlorophyll to convert carbon dioxide and water into carbohydrate, taking in sunlight as an energy source for the reaction (*photosynthesis*). This reaction is the reverse of the one we use to generate energy by burning glucose.

Daily requirement: the RDA value for magnesium is 300 to 350 mg for an adult, with higher amounts (400 to 450 mg) for teenagers or pregnant and lactating women.

As magnesium salts are much more soluble than those of calcium, absorption from the intestine is more efficient. High-fibre diets increase the excretion of magnesium (and most other minerals) through the faeces. Water loss through vomiting, diarrhoea, sweating, or the use of diuretics, all decrease the body's supply of magnesium (and other water-soluble minerals).

Food sources: the richest food sources are nuts (including peanuts, a legume), cereal grains and fish.

100 g (3½ oz) of peanuts provide 170 mg of magnesium; almonds, walnuts and brazil nuts all contain slightly more than this: 60 to 70 mg of magnesium per 30 g (1 oz). Whole-grain cereals (including brown rice) provide 30 to 50 mg of magnesium in a 30 g (1 oz) serving and 100 to 150 mg/100 g (3½ oz). A typical 90 g (3 oz) serving of tuna contains

20 mg of magnesium, while the same portion of tinned salmon gives 30 mg.

Although all green plants contain chlorophyll, this is not a particularly rich dietary source of the mineral. The magnesium atom is locked in the middle of a ring structure (*porphyrin*) and it is difficult for the body to extract the magnesium from this.

Dolomite, a carbonate of calcium and magnesium, is a popular form of dietary supplement. Epsom salts (magnesium sulphate) are less commonly used nowadays.

Symptoms of deficiency or excess: a deficiency of magnesium is accompanied by nausea, muscle spasms and tremors, lethargy, apathy and behavioural problems. The addition of magnesium to the diet resolves these problems in otherwise healthy individuals.

There are no known symptoms of magnesium excess.

CALCIUM

Metabolism: there is more calcium in the body than any other mineral element – about 2 per cent of body weight. This means that a person weighing 64 kg (10 stone) will have more than 1 kg (2¼ lb) of calcium in his body. Almost all of this is in the bones and teeth as the carbonate and phosphate. Of the 10 mg/100 ml calcium circulating in blood serum, about 4.5 mg occurs as free calcium ions; the remainder is combined with protein.

Another important use of calcium in the body is the way it assists in the action of blood clotting. Like sodium and potassium, it is involved in nerve impulse transmission (by stimulating the release of *acetylcholine*) and in stimulating muscle contraction. The presence of calcium is also necessary for the absorption of vitamin B12 from the intestine, where a complex is formed between calcium, the vitamin, and a protein secreted by the stomach.

If the level of blood calcium (normally about 10 mg/100 ml) is high, a hormone from the thyroid gland inhibits its release from bone tissue. If blood calcium is low, a hormone from the parathyroid glands, together with vitamin D, increases the release of calcium from bone into the blood and decreases excretion by the kidney.

Daily requirement: normal healthy adults need to absorb about 800 mg of calcium daily (US value), which increases to about 1.2 g daily for teenage children and pregnant or lactating women. The UK recommended daily intake is 500 mg for adults.

Food sources: one of the best dietary sources of calcium is milk, which contains 775 mg per 600 ml (1 pint). The calcium is carried through to butter and cheese: full-fat cheese has about 7 mg/g; cottage cheese, however, has less than one-tenth of this amount.

For vegans, or those who have an allergy to milk, or Orientals for whom milk has never formed a significant part of the diet, hard or mineral water are good dietary sources. Calcium is added to white bread, but it is not present to any significant extent in wholemeal bread. Watercress, soya and brewer's yeast (each with about 200 mg/100 g) are the best alternative food sources. But without dairy products, you really need a tablet supplement to get adequate calcium in a form which can be easily absorbed.

Absorption: vitamin D and lactose both increase the absorption of calcium. Calcium salts are more soluble in acid solutions, and therefore they dissolve in acidic gastric juice and are absorbed into the upper part of the small intestine before the digestive juices become too alkaline.

There are some foods that contain compounds which form insoluble salts with calcium and hence prevent its absorption. Spinach and rhubarb, for example, contain *oxalic acid*, and calcium oxalate is insoluble. However, clinical studies have failed to show any calcium depletion in children given oxalic acid diets under controlled conditions.

In the bran of whole-wheat grains there is a substance called *phytic acid*, which forms insoluble calcium phytate with calcium salts. This insolubility would prevent calcium absorption. When we eat bread, this factor is not important since an enzyme (*phytase*) is added during baking to react chemically with the phytic acid so that the product of its reaction with calcium is soluble and therefore accessible to the body.

The insolubility of calcium phytate should be important when whole-grain cereals are eaten, but no depletion of blood calcium has been detected in such a diet. Perhaps the excess of calcium in the milk which usually accompanies cereals when they are eaten compensates for that which is lost.

Dietary fibre contributes to loss of calcium as of many other minerals. Clinical studies have shown a direct link between increased fibre intake and decreased blood calcium. For those on a high-fibre diet, extra calcium intake is recommended.

Calcium is also lost through sweating and urinary excretion, as well as in faeces. However, unlike the case of sodium and potassium excretion, where sweat and urine losses are compensated in the body, there is no compensating mechanism for calcium.

Symptoms of deficiency or excess: a deficiency of calcium causes bone disorders which, in the extreme case, may develop into softening of the bone (*osteomalacia*) or reduction of the mass of the bone (*osteoporosis*), but these are found mostly in the elderly or those suffering from general malnutrition.

Excess calcium intake is not known to cause any ill effects – not even in conditions such as arthritis or kidney stones, where calcium may be important, although sufferers from these complaints would be well advised to limit calcium in their diet.

IRON

Metabolism: although it is widely distributed in the body, our overall iron content is relatively small. A 64 kg (10 stone) adult has between 2 and 4 g of iron, about two-thirds of which is in the form of haemoglobin, the red colouring matter in blood cells. Much of the remaining iron in the blood stream is bound to a protein (*transferritin*), the sole purpose of which is to transport iron around the body.

The role of haemoglobin in the red blood cells is to carry oxygen from the lungs to the tissues. Mammals have evolved with an iron-containing molecule to do this job, and there are other animals that have a cobalt-bound protein or vanadium-bound protein for this purpose. Neither of these elements can carry oxygen as efficiently as iron, however, and hence all the higher animals have an iron-bound oxygen carrier.

The iron is situated at the centre of a large chemical structure (*porphyrin*) to form a molecule called haem. The protein (*globin*) is wrapped around it to form a complex protein. There are four haems in every molecule of haemoglobin. When oxygen is absorbed and subsequently released, the globin 'breathes' out and in to accommodate the oxygen within it. Some 95 per cent of the oxygen in our bodies is carried in this way; the other 5 per cent simply dissolves in the water of our blood plasma.

About one-third of the carbon dioxide we exhale is also carried around the blood stream by haemoglobin. The rest of the carbon dioxide also dissolves in the water of the blood plasma.

Iron in haem is also a part of many enzymes (*cytochromes*) which are used to carry electrical charges around the body, both positive (*proton*) and negative (*electron*).

Daily requirement: the dietary requirement for iron is in the range 10 to 20 mg daily, though the amount we need to absorb daily is only 1 to 2 mg. Women need more than men because of the monthly blood loss in menstruation.

Some women who take iron supplements find that they cause constipation. The answer is to try different preparations: some will produce this effect, others won't.

If you are taking iron to make up menstrual losses, you should stop taking the tablets two or three days before the period and begin again forty-eight hours after bleeding has stopped. Taking the tablets during the period generally increases menstrual flow. If you recommence taking tablets as the bleeding tails off, this may restart the flow for a further day or so.

Food sources: the richest food sources of iron are red meat and offal, but there are many other foods which contain iron in significant amounts, especially dark green, leafy vegetables and whole-grain cereals.

Kidneys and liver contain 7 to 8 mg/100 g, but beef, lamb, pork and ham only 1 to 2 mg/100 g. Dry brewer's yeast is one of the richest non-meat sources with 17.5 mg/100 g, but whereas eating 100 g (3½ oz) of meat is practicable, taking that amount of brewer's yeast is not. Haricot beans have 6.5 mg/100 g, but most beans and peanuts have only 1 to 3 mg/100 g.

Breakfast cereals have natural iron in them and this is often supplemented. For vegetarians and vegans, this is probably the most accessible source of iron in the diet. Bran-enriched wheat flakes contain about 40 mg/100 g, so the normal 30 g (1 oz) serving provides the whole day's supply. Other cereals will supply 3 to 8 mg of iron in a generous (50 g/1¾ oz) portion. Most fish, milk and dairy products are poor in iron. So are most fruits; notable exceptions are dried figs, prunes or apricots, which contain 3 to 4 mg/100 g. One egg contains about 1 mg of iron, mostly in the yolk.

Absorption: one problem that has to be considered in assessing iron intake is its availability for absorption into the body. Several studies suggest that as little as 10 per cent of the iron we eat is actually absorbed. Iron from meat is more readily absorbed by the body than iron from plant sources. Furthermore, the presence of meat in the diet assists the absorption of plant iron.

The presence of vitamin C improves the absorption of iron, particularly that from plant sources. The tannin in tea and the fibre in whole-grain bread and cereals inhibit iron absorption. So we need 10 to 20 mg per day in our diet to be sure of absorbing the 1 to 2 mg daily that is required for metabolism.

Apart from the iron in our diet which passes through the body without absorption, we excrete another 0.5 mg or so daily in the bile pigments (like *bilirubin*) which give the dark colour to the faeces. Only a small amount is lost in urine.

The main losses of iron from the body occur by blood donation or bleeding, whether through accident or menstruation. In these cases, or if you have a low vitamin C or high tea or fibre intake, or are a vegetarian or vegan, iron tablet supplements are desirable. Otherwise they should not be necessary.

Symptoms of deficiency or excess: a deficiency of iron generally shows itself as anaemia – insufficient oxygen-carrying red blood cells. The symptoms are fatigue, lethargy, dizziness, insomnia, headaches, high pulse rate and palpitations.

Even without reaching the stage of obvious anaemia, low blood iron levels are said to be associated with greater virulence of oral, bronchial and gastric infections. This state occurs because the body has insufficient iron to form the enzymes which mobilize the white blood cells that fight infectious diseases.

An excess of iron in the diet causes deposition of the element in the tissues of the body, first in the liver, then in the heart and pancreas. The result is a condition known as *haemochromatosis*. For this to occur you would normally need something in the range of 50 to 100 mg of iron daily, which is difficult to achieve in a normal diet without supplements. But the message is: don't take iron supplements unless advised to do so by your doctor, or you feel from the above discussion that some *small* additional doses might be beneficial.

ZINC

Metabolism: zinc is found in relatively high concentrations in the eye, though why this should be so isn't known. The main function of the element in the body is participating in important enzyme reactions, like the conversion of bicarbonate into carbon dioxide and water; the first stage of the detoxification of alcohol; and in protein digestion. Zinc also activates insulin and thus plays a part in carbohydrate metabolism.

It's been mentioned before that some atoms move around the body in groups, but without a positive or negative electrical charge; these are called *radicals*. The body appears to need a limited supply of radicals for normal healthy biochemistry, particularly in fighting disease. If we get an excess of them, however, they seem to promote disease, especially cancer. The concentration of radicals must, therefore, be regulated carefully. This job is carried out in animals and humans by special metal-containing proteins: in humans, the metals involved are zinc and copper.

In fact, there are more than seventy enzymes in all that require zinc, either as a component or as an activator (*cofactor*). Only a little zinc appears to be absorbed, however, through the intestinal wall. As with iron, what there is in the body is used and recycled.

Daily requirement: the RDA value for zinc in adults is 15 mg. The total body content is over 2 g, located mainly in the eyes, sex glands and hair.

Food sources: zinc is another of those minerals which is widespread in plants but which is in a form that is not readily accessible to humans. Once again, it appears that the fibre and phytic acid in plants inhibit absorption (see page 172).

Zinc is found in a wide range of food, the richest sources being meat, poultry, fish, eggs, milk and dairy products, and whole-grain cereals. It is so widespread that even with minimal absorption there is little difficulty in getting an adequate supply on a varied diet.

Symptoms of deficiency or excess: zinc deficiency in humans is well known. It produces retarded growth and development, poor wound healing, and low resistance to infection. Zinc has long been used in the form of its oxide or carbonate (calamine) to treat skin rashes, insect bites or cuts – it's a safe and simple remedy. It may be that part of its action at least is through local absorption into the body. Poor vitamin A metabolism may also be associated with zinc deficiency.

As with some other minerals and vitamins, steroid medication (cortisol for arthritis, or contraceptive pills), or high alcohol intake inhibit zinc absorption.

Symptoms of zinc toxicity have not been defined.

COPPER

Metabolism: the normal body content of copper is about 120 mg. It is absorbed from food in the intestine and carried around in the blood by chemical binding to a protein. As this protein is involved in the body's use of iron, copper seems to be necessary for the normal formation of haemoglobin and the prevention of anaemia.

Copper is an activator (*cofactor*) or constituent of a number of enzymes. It is involved in the conversion of the amino acid tyrosine to the pigment melanin, which gives colour to our hair and skin. Copper forms a complex with other proteins to provide enzymes involved in respiratory oxidation, and copper enzymes are also necessary for the formation of connective tissue in our skin, and cartilage in our joints. This may provide the physiological basis for the folk remedy of wearing copper bracelets to ease arthritis. Copper also reduces the risk of gastric bleeding from the administration of aspirin to arthritics. For the role of copper in controlling radicals in the body, see page 175.

Daily requirement: no definite value for copper intake has been established, but it seems that 2 mg per day is adequate for health.

Food sources: liver and lobster are the best food sources of copper (up to 12 mg/100 g). Vegetarians can get their supply from dry brewer's yeast, nuts and whole-wheat cereals (up to 4 mg/100 g).

Soft water or a water supply derived from the increasingly widespread acid rain will dissolve more copper from water pipes than hard water. Acid rain is produced when raindrops dissolve gases from heavy industrial emissions. These industries discharge significant quantities of the oxides of sulphur, nitrogen and carbon into the air, and when they are dissolved in water, these form sulphuric, nitric and carbonic acids respectively.

In Britain acid rain becomes more of a problem the further north you go, for a number of reasons. There is more heavy industry concentrated in the north; lower temperatures further north mean more coal fires producing more gases; prevailing south-westerly winds carry noxious emissions in a northerly and easterly direction across the country; and there is a greater rainfall in the more mountainous regions, which are also located to the north (and west) of the country. Water run-off is also more acidic from the igneous and metamorphic rocks of the north and the west, than that collected from the largely chalk uplands of the south and east.

If you live in the north of England in a modern house with copper water pipes, you will almost certainly get more than enough copper in your drinking water alone, far more than you are likely to get from your food, whatever your diet.

In Europe and North America, because of the greater land masses and distribution of heavy industry, acid rain is more widespread. In Europe it tends to be concentrated in Scandinavia (because of the prevailing winds and rainfall) and Germany (because of the amount of heavy industry). For some people in these countries, copper poisoning from acid rain is already a problem.

Symptoms of deficiency or excess: though not widespread, copper deficiency is occasionally observed, mainly in infants. Milk – even breast milk – is low in copper, so babies are born with enough copper to last them for a few months until they move on to a solid diet. If this is also largely milk- and cereal-based, copper deficiency may develop, with symptoms resembling those of anaemia (see page 175) or scurvy (see page 160).

Copper poisoning, formerly a rare condition, is becoming more common due to increasing industrialization (see above). Extra copper in the body is deposited first in the liver and brain, causing trembling, slurred speech, poor co-ordination, neurosis and muscle tension. Changes in behaviour with a tendency towards depression and psychotic reactions may be the first symptoms.

COBALT

Metabolism: cobalt is a constituent of vitamin B12; this appears to be its only function in the human body. The vitamin is used in the manufacture of haemoglobin, so cobalt is important in the prevention of anaemia.

In clinical trials, administration of cobalt salts has produced increased manufacture of red blood cells by healthy individuals. There is evidently some physiological pathway for B12 synthesis, but just what this is isn't known yet. Some authorities maintain that no such pathway exists, and that we must ingest vitamin B12 as such in our diet, but cobalt is unlikely to increase the generation of red blood cells in any way other than through vitamin B12. It was less than three decades ago that the chemical structure of vitamin B12 was determined, so research into the physiological role of cobalt is still at an early stage.

Daily requirement: the requirement for cobalt in the diet is not known. What information there is suggests that as little as 10 to 15 mcg daily is adequate for health.

Food sources: little is known also of the cobalt content of foods because it occurs in such small quantities. It is found as cobalt salts in vegetables and as vitamin B12, the principal dietary source, in meat, eggs, milk and dairy produce.

Symptoms of deficiency or excess: no symptoms have yet been recorded for either an excess or deficiency of cobalt. It is not as widespread in nature as many of the other heavy metals already discussed, nor is it used in industry as widely – mainly for making types of steel, and for the blue pigments in glass and pottery. Its use is so specialized that cobalt poisoning from environmental pollution or other excess ingestion is rare.

Because we need so little cobalt daily, vegetarians generally get sufficient in vegetables, milk and eggs. Vegans, eating only cereals and vegetables, may develop deficiency states, since what little cobalt there is in these foods is almost entirely in the form of salts, not as B12, and these are not as effective a source of the element. Brewer's yeast supplies a little cobalt as the vitamin, but a supplement is advisable for vegans.

CHROMIUM

Metabolism: chromium is needed for reactions involving insulin in the metabolism of sugar and fat. It lowers the time required for blood sugar to return to its normal level after a fasting person takes a drink of sugar and water only. This is known as the glucose tolerance test. The time lag

for blood sugar to return to normal is generally about two and a ha
hours.

Diabetics taking insulin absorb more chromium than health
individuals. The normal body content is about 1.5 mg.

There is some evidence also that chromium assists in other aspects o
the metabolism of lipids, lowers blood pressure, and prevent
hypertension. Some researchers have therefore inferred that it slow
down the ageing process.

Daily requirement: no daily requirement has been established fo
chromium, but 200 to 300 mcg per day seems to be adequate for health

Food sources: chromium is found most abundantly in whole-grair
cereals, dry brewer's yeast and cheese. Shrimps, lobster, butter, meat anc
mushrooms have lower but still significant amounts.

Chromium exists in food in two forms: in a poorly absorbed inorganic
form and as a more readily assimilated organic complex. The latter may
be sold in health supplies stores as GTF (glucose tolerance factor)
chromium, in which the metal is bound to niacin and several amino
acids; it is extracted from brewer's yeast. While the body absorbs only
some 1 per cent of the inorganic chromium in the diet it may absorb 10 to
20 per cent of the organically bound form. Relative amounts of the two
types in various foods, and how these affect overall absorption, have not
yet been assessed.

Symptoms of deficiency or excess: apart from its role in lowering blood
sugar and blood lipid, little is known about chromium metabolism, so
neither deficiency nor excess states have yet been defined.

MANGANESE

Metabolism: the normal body content of manganese is 12 to 15 mg. It is
distributed in all tissues but is concentrated in the liver, skin, bones and
muscles. Most of it is carried around the body bound to a protein.

Manganese is an activator (*cofactor*) of many enzymes; it is actually a
constituent of some of them. Protein synthesis, fatty-acid metabolism,
carbohydrate metabolism, bone development, and the production of
defence mechanisms against disease all require manganese. Arthritics and
diabetics tend to have low blood manganese levels.

Daily requirement: the exact amount of manganese we need in our diets
has not yet been determined. Studies suggest that an intake of 5 to 10 mg
daily is adequate.

Food sources: the best food sources of manganese are whole-grain cereals, pulses, nuts (including peanuts) and avocado pears, all of which contain some 2 to 4 mg/100 g of food. Tea is also a rich source of the mineral. Meat, fish, fruit, milk and dairy products are generally poor sources.

Symptoms of deficiency or excess: symptoms of manganese deficiency have not yet been recorded in human beings. Manganese is involved in so many of the body's chemical reactions that its presence in the diet is certainly essential, but as it is quite widespread and the daily requirement is small, deficiency states are unlikely. Those suffering from diabetes or arthritis may benefit from tablet supplements, but under no circumstances should you exceed 10 mg daily until more is known of manganese biochemistry.

Manganese excess is similarly rarely encountered, except in those who work at processing the metal from its ores. Then, the effects are most visible in nervous disorder: difficulty in walking and speaking, and involuntary movements of muscles of the hands and face.

MOLYBDENUM

Metabolism: molybdenum is found in the body as a constituent of three enzymes which fulfil many different biochemical functions.

Daily requirement: the dietary requirement of molybdenum is not yet known, but amounts up to 500 mcg daily have been found adequate for good health.

Food sources: molybdenum is widely distributed in foods: whole-grain cereals, legumes (including peanuts), offal (like kidneys and liver) and some dark green, leafy vegetables.

Symptoms of deficiency or excess: no deficiency or toxicity states have been observed for molybdenum, so there is no evidence to suggest any need for tablet supplementation.

PHOSPHORUS

Metabolism: phosphorus is found as a component of the membrane wall of every cell in the body, primarily as phospholipids. In addition, a phosphorus compound (ATP) is one of the body's main energy carriers. Calcium phosphate and calcium carbonate together make up two-thirds of the substance of our bones and teeth, and this is where most of the phosphorus in our bodies (about 80 per cent) is located.

The nucleic acids (*DNA* and *RNA*), so called because they are located at the centres or nuclei of our cells, contain phosphorus. It is the nucleic acids in sperm and ovum cells that carry the genetic message or blueprint which determines the character of our offspring.

Many compounds have a phosphate group tacked on to them as the first stage of a chain reaction which constitutes metabolism of that substance. No system in the body can function without phosphorus. We have about 600 g in our bodies (about 1 per cent of our body weight).

Absorption of phosphorus from the diet is highly effective. About 70 per cent of the amount we ingest is taken up by the small intestine. Unlike metallic elements, which are excreted mainly in the faeces, phosphorus (as the phosphate ion) is excreted in the urine. The excretion rate is controlled by hormones of the parathyroid glands located in the neck.

Daily requirement: the RDA for phosphorus is 800 mg, the same as for calcium. However, we do not encounter the same absorption problems with phosphorus as with calcium and the heavy metals.

Food sources: all high-protein foods are rich in phosphorus: meat, fish, milk and dairy products, eggs, nuts and whole-grain cereals. Some of the phosphorus in cereals is not available to the body as it is chemically bound up as phytin.

A normal 150 g (5¼ oz) portion of lean beef or haddock provides 350 mg of phosphorus – nearly half the day's requirement. The same weight of peanuts would give you 600 mg of phosphorus, but this is much more than one would normally eat at one sitting. 90 g (3 oz) of salmon (half a medium-size tin) has 250 mg of phosphorus; 90 g (3 oz) of tuna, 200 mg. One medium-size egg contains only 80 mg of phosphorus.

There is 300 mg of phosphorus in 250 ml (½ pint) of milk. Full-fat cheese has about 150 mg per 30 g (1 oz), but cottage cheese contains only about one-third of this amount.

If you have worked through all these sections on vitamins and minerals, you will have noticed by now that in taking away the fat (cream) of milk to prepare cottage cheese, most of the nutrients are taken away as well – the nutrients we expect to derive from dairy produce. This is illustrated in Table 9.

From this table you can see that although we take in fewer calories in cottage cheese compared to full-fat cheese, we have lost nearly half of the protein, most of the calcium, phosphorus and vitamin A, and some of the potassium as well. All of this applies to cottage cheese retaining 1 to 2 per cent fat. In the uncreamed variety, the nutrient value is even lower. Cottage cheese is, in fact, 80 per cent water. This makes its food value very low. It would be better for slimmers to eat less of the whole-fat or medium-fat cheeses and get the nutrients along with the fat.

Table 9 Comparison of the main nutrients in equal weights (28 g/1 oz) of full-fat cheese and low-fat (1 to 2 per cent) cottage cheese

	Weight (g)	Energy (kcal)	Protein (g)	Carbohydrate (g)	Saturated fat (g)	Unsaturated fat (g)	Water (g)	Calcium (mg)	Phosphorus (mg)	Potassium (mg)	Vitamin A (mcg)
full-fat cheese	28	115	7	trace	6	2.5	12	204	145	28	90
cottage cheese	28	22	4	1	0.3	trace	22.5	19	40	25[1]	4.5

Quantity of nutrients in cottage cheese expressed as an approximate ratio to those in full-fat cheese

	Weight (g)	Energy (kcal)	Protein (g)	Carbohydrate (g)	Saturated fat (g)	Unsaturated fat (g)	Water (g)	Calcium (mg)	Phosphorus (mg)	Potassium (mg)	Vitamin A (mcg)
full-fat cheese	1	1	1	1	1	1	1	1	1	1	1
cottage cheese	1	1/6	1/2	100?[2]	1/20	trace	2	1/10	1/3	1	1/20

Notes
1 This figure is for low-fat cottage cheese. Uncreamed cottage cheese has only 9 g of potassium per 28 g (1 oz).
2 As there is only a trace of carbohydrate in full-fat cheese, the ratio of that in cottage cheese:full-fat cheese can only be estimated very approximately.

Symptoms of deficiency or excess: because phosphorus is so widely distributed in foods, deficiency, even amongst vegetarians and vegans, is rare. Conversely, because it is used in so many body reactions, and easily excreted through the kidneys, toxic excesses are never encountered.

SULPHUR

Metabolism: sulphur, like phosphorus, is a constituent of every cell in our bodies. It is a part of three of the twenty or so common amino acids (*cystine, cysteine* and *methionine*) and, therefore, finds its way into the body's proteins and cellular lipoproteins.

Sulphur is also a component of two of the vitamins of the B complex (*thiamin* and *biotin*). It is one of the elements in insulin (the pancreatic hormone) and is a part of an important enzyme activator (*coenzyme A*). Combined with oxygen it forms the sulphate ion, which is the second most abundant negative ion in the fluid inside cells (*intracellular fluid*).

Daily requirement: because sulphur is so widespread in foods, no daily requirement level has been established.

Food sources: as sulphur is a component of amino acids, it is found along with phosphorus in high-protein foods: meat, fish, milk and dairy produce, nuts, eggs and whole-grain cereals.

The sulphur in our diet comes mainly from this protein, with smaller amounts from sulphates in mineral waters and food additives, and as sulphur dioxide (E220), which is used extensively as a bleaching agent and preservative in food preparation. As a result of the chemical action of sulphur dioxide, treated foods may contain sulphites which are known to cause hypersensitivity or allergic responses in asthmatics.

Symptoms of deficiency or excess: no symptoms of either deficiency or excess have been defined but, as explained above, hypersensitivity reactions to sulphur in food additives are reported to be quite common.

SELENIUM

Metabolism: the normal body content of selenium is about 20 mg. It is a component of an enzyme which is used in the body to break down the products of lipid oxidation and to remove toxins from the blood.

There is some suggestion that selenium might be complementary to vitamin E in some of its actions, and that it can replace sulphur (which it resembles chemically) in certain tissues, but this is still hypothetical. It has not even been established yet whether selenium works with vitamin E or as an alternative in its role as antioxidant.

Breast cancer has been correlated statistically with low selenium levels, but it is not certain that this correlation has any significance. No causal relationship has been established. However, other studies have linked breast cancer with a diet high in saturated fat, so as selenium is involved in lipid metabolism, a link between breast cancer and body selenium levels is plausible.

Daily requirement: no requirement has been established for selenium, but a daily intake of 150 mcg has been tentatively suggested as the correct desirable level.

Food sources: most of our selenium comes originally from plants. There is great variation in the soil content of selenium and therefore in the plants grown in these soils and in the animals that graze there. The best food sources of selenium are meat, milk, eggs, fish and whole-grain cereals, which may contain up to 20 mcg/100 g.

Symptoms of deficiency or excess: animals are known to suffer symptoms of selenium deficiency but this has not been reliably reported in humans, even in Finland, where the soil contains very little selenium. At the present time there is no biochemical basis for the use of selenium tablet supplements.

Some evidence of selenium poisoning in humans has been suggested with production of tooth and gum disorders, but because the quantities of the mineral involved are so small, definite links have not yet been established. Selenium is undoubtedly highly toxic, however, and under no circumstances should your daily intake exceed 300 mcg, that is, double the level thought desirable for optimal health.

Selenium is a common ingredient of medicated hair shampoos; how much is absorbed from this source through the skin and hair isn't known. Selenium is also used in many xerographic photocopying processes, and those who operate such machines for extended periods may well absorb significant quantities.

FLUORINE

Metabolism: fluorine occurs in the body as the negatively charged fluoride ion. It is absorbed from the intestine, and excesses are excreted by the kidneys. It is incorporated into the structure of teeth and bones: it appears to increase the resistance of teeth to decay and gives strength to our bones, especially during childhood and in old age. In particular, softening of the bones of the inner ear, leading to progressively increased deafness, has been found to be arrested and reversed by administration of fluoride. It is not true to say that fluoride is of no use to the body after puberty. It is incorporated into the structure of our bones throughout life; this has been unequivocally established.

Fluorine atoms can be stacked compactly with calcium in a solid crystal structure, so the two elements are often found together in geological minerals (*apatite* and *fluorspar*) as well as in our bones. These provide a natural source of fluorine in water supplies.

In addition to protecting our teeth and bones, there is some evidence now that fluorine inhibits calcification of the arteries, though the mechanism for this action is not known.

Daily requirement: no level of fluoride has yet been established as optimal for health, but up to 5 mg per day for adults is regarded as beneficial. There are 2 to 3 g of fluoride in an adult body.

Food sources: seafood and tea are the main sources of fluoride, containing up to 15 and 100 parts per million respectively. These provide far more fluoride for most people, especially for avid strong-tea drinkers, than is likely to come from the water itself, whether or not it has been artificially fluoridated.

Water supplies in Britain and the US are now frequently fluoridated to a level of one part per million (1 mg/litre). On an adult daily intake of 2 l (3½ pints) of water, this amounts to 2 mg per day. Naturally fluoridated water may contain up to 6 ppm, though concentrations are usually much less than this. These levels would correspond to an intake of up to 12 mg of fluoride daily just from drinking water. Whatever fluoride we get from our drinking water, we take in up to another 4 mg daily from tea or solid food.

The tablets given to children to protect their teeth usually contain just over 2 mg of sodium fluoride (1 mg of fluoride in each).

Fluoride levels cannot become concentrated in water when there is a high level of calcium or magnesium present, as in hard-water districts. This is because the metal ions join together with the fluoride to form insoluble calcium fluoride or magnesium fluoride.

There is absolutely no chemical difference between the fluoride which is added artificially to water supplies and that which occurs naturally. In salts of this type, the metal part and the fluoride part have a more or less independent existence once they are dissolved in water.

Symptoms of deficiency or excess: deficiency of fluoride predisposes us to dental decay and brittle bones, especially in growing children and in the elderly. One of the first and most obvious symptoms of fluoride excess is mottling of the teeth, which may be unsightly but in itself is harmless.

There is little doubt about the beneficial effects of low concentrations of fluoride. Fluorine may not be an essential mineral element, but it is so widespread in nature that it is found universally in the human body.

In high concentration fluoride is certainly toxic. Evidence has been found recently that it interferes with the chemical links (*hydrogen bonds*) that hold together the long spiral chains of bio-organic polymers like proteins and nucleic acids. No direct physiological significance of these chemical findings has yet been established, but this may be the mechanism by which fluoride interferes with joint and nerve biochemistry. It is conceivable also that if fluoride gets into the cell it could attack the RNA and DNA strands in the nucleus by this same mechanism and thus cause cancer or genetic defects.

In order to produce those damaging effects, we would need high concentrations of fluoride: just how high has not been established, but fluoride toxicity or fluorosis has never been reported in people who drink water with less than 4 ppm of fluoride.

People living all their lives in areas with a natural water fluoride content of 2 ppm (and hence taking up to 4 mg per day from this source alone) have shown no signs of fluorosis at post mortem.

Also, doses of up to 70 mg daily of sodium fluoride (containing 32.5 mg of fluoride) have been used to treat cases of bone disease (like osteoporosis) without any signs of fluoride toxicity.

More than 30 million people in the US have been drinking artificially fluoridated water for more than a quarter of a century with only beneficial results (*except* where they have a high fluoride intake from some other source).

On the other hand, in the Punjab region of India, where the inhabitants continually have an extremely high level of fluoride intake, there is widespread evidence of bone changes and joint and nerve disorders.

When fluoride levels build up in the blood, first of all more is excreted by the kidneys. As calcium and magnesium fluorides are only sparingly soluble in water and the concentration of calcium and magnesium ions in the blood is more than a hundred times that of fluoride, these metals remove fluoride for deposit in the teeth and bones. This has been shown experimentally with many people.

The overwhelming balance of evidence indicates that water fluoride concentrations of up to 10 ppm (representing a total intake of 15 to 20 mg per day) are not harmful in the short term and do produce considerable beneficial effects throughout life, not only in the young. Because long-term effects are not yet established, recommended intake is kept down to 1 ppm in water and 5 mg per day total allowance, though it is fairly certain that in this there is a considerable safety margin.

Fluoridation of water supplies does decrease dental decay and does increase bone strength throughout life. It should not be regarded, however, as an easy alternative to sensible diet control in the young. The main cause of tooth decay in children is almost certainly frequent eating of sweets and infrequent brushing of teeth. Even water fluoridation will not completely offset the damage that these practices cause. Quite apart from causing dental decay, the high sugar intake leads to obesity and probably contributes to diabetes and heart and circulatory diseases. Education not fluoridation is the only satisfactory answer to this problem.

The chief objection to fluoridation is not that it shouldn't be used as an easy option for prevention of tooth decay: it isn't. Nor that is causes illness: at these concentrations it prevents more disease than it provokes. Nor that it infringes human rights: civilized society has all sorts of food legislation to protect the population as a whole. The main problem with artificial water fluoridation is the lack of control. No potentially toxic substance should ever be administered without strict controls. In summer, manual workers or sportsmen may drink several times the normal daily fluid intake, either as water or beer. If they also drink strong tea, there is a very real chance that they may get close to what is regarded as the safe upper limit of fluoride intake. Until the long-term effects are known this is a possibility we should avoid.

CHLORINE

Metabolism: chlorine is an element which behaves chemically in many ways like fluorine. It is also a poisonous gas, as is fluorine, but in the body it is found in the form of the harmless negatively charged chloride ion.

It is a major constituent of the fluid that surrounds our cells (*extracellular fluid*) and is found also in gastric juice, which is largely hydrochloric acid. It works with sodium and potassium in regulating the salt/water balance of the body.

Like fluoride and phosphate, it is readily absorbed by the intestine and excreted by the kidneys.

Daily requirement: no daily requirement for chloride has been defined.

Food sources: the main food source is salt, sodium chloride, which is found naturally in meat, seafood, celery and other foods. Our intake is complemented by the amount of salt we add in food preparation. A normal mixed diet contains enough salt for our needs, but vegans will find it more difficult to get adequate amounts as they exclude meat and fish. Celery, beet and dandelion greens, spinach and kale are the vegetable sources most abundant in sodium chloride.

Symptoms of deficiency or excess: deficiency of salt is rarely a problem (see page 167). Chloride is ingested almost exclusively as salt, and the symptoms of excess are those due to the sodium rather than the chloride.

IODINE

Metabolism: the only known role of iodine in the body is as a part of the thyroid hormone *thyroxine*. This is essential for the control of the rate of the body's metabolic reactions. Secretion of thyroxine is itself under the control of the master endocrine gland (*pituitary gland*), which is located at the base of the brain.

Iodine is absorbed almost 100 per cent into the blood stream from the stomach and intestine. Using one of its proteins, the thyroid gland successively adds up to four iodine atoms to the amino acid *tyrosine*. Once there are three or four iodine atoms on tyrosine, the resulting compound is also active as a thyroid hormone alongside thyroxine.

Daily requirement: the daily requirement for iodine is 1 mcg/kg of body weight, or about 60 mcg daily for a 64 kg (10 stone) adult. The RDA figures are about twice this amount, giving a margin of safety to prevent deficiency states.

Food sources: iodine is not widespread in foods. Seafood (but not fresh-water fish) is the best source. Iodine is often added to salt to ensure that we get an adequate supply, in view of the amount of salt that is used in cooking. Certain cultures use seaweed in their diet, and this is a good source too. Eggs may contain iodine if the hens have been fed meal derived from kelp. In some countries, iodate (a radical containing iodine and oxygen) is added to the dough in bread-making, possibly providing another source.

Iodine is a disinfectant. When it is used in dairies for this purpose, it may pass along the food chain into the milk. It is sometimes used instead of chlorine to disinfect drinking water.

Some foods contain a substance called *progoitrin* which is changed by enzyme action into a compound that prevents our bodies making thyroxine from iodine. Progoitrin is found in the seeds and edible portions of the mustard family – turnips, cabbage, cauliflower, cress and kale – but fortunately it is inactivated when the food is cooked. If significant quantities of these foods are eaten raw, they will inhibit thyroxine formation; they should be avoided by people with thyroid disorders.

Symptoms of deficiency or excess: deficiency of iodine, and thence of thyroxine, leads to enlargement of the thyroid gland and production of the condition known as goitre: in an extreme case, the throat becomes enlarged and the eyes protrude. The condition is reversible over weeks or months by administration of iodine in the diet.

Up to ten times the RDA value of iodine may be consumed without ill effects. The thyroid gland stores some of this and the surplus is excreted in urine.

FURTHER READING

The following books are listed by subject in alphabetical order, as are the authors within each subject division. The contents of most of these books should be accessible to a general readership, though some of them are technical and some of them popular in their level of presentation.

Acupuncture

Macdonald, A., *Acupuncture: From ancient art to modern medicine*, Allen & Unwin, 1982
Mann, F., *Scientific Aspects of Acupuncture*, Heinemann, 1977
Marcus, P., *Acupuncture*, Thorsons, 1984

Allergy

Bright, M., *Living With Your Allergy*, Granada, 1982
Bucst, R., *Food Intolerance: What it is and how to cope with it*, Prism Alpha, 1984
Davies, G. H., *Overcoming Food Allergies*, Ashgrove Press, 1985
Dickenson, D., *How to Strengthen Your Immune System*, Arlington Press, 1984
Eagle, R., *Eating and Allergy*, Futura, 1979
　　　　Allergies, Hamlyn, 1980
Hanssen, M., *E for Additives*, Thorsons, 1984
Mackarness, R., *Eating Dangerously: The hazards of hidden allergies*, Harcourt Brace Jovanovich, 1976
　　　　Not All in the Mind, Pan, 1976
　　　　Chemical Victims, Pan, 1980
Mumby, K., *The Food Allergy Plan*, Unwin, 1985
Randolph, T. G. and Moss, R. W., *Allergies*, Thorsons, 1984
Rippere, V., *The Allergy Problem*, Thorsons, 1983
Workman, E., Hunter, J. and Jones, V. Alun, *The Allergy Diet*, Martin Dunitz, 1984

Alternative medicine – general

Eagle, R., *A Guide to Alternative Medicine*, BBC Publications, 1980
Fulder, S., *The Handbook of Complementary Medicine*, Coronet, 1984
Hill, A. (ed.), *A Visual Encyclopedia of Unconventional Medicine*, New English Library, 1979

Stanway, A., *Alternative Medicine: A guide to natural therapies*, MacDonald and Jane's, 1980

Biochemistry

Campbell, P. N. and Smith, A. O., *Biochemistry*, Churchill Livingstone, 1982
Pickering, W. R. and Wood, E. J., *Introducing Biochemistry*, Murray, 1982
Rafelson, M. E., *Basic Biochemistry*, Macmillan, 1982
Stryer, L., *Biochemistry*, W. H. Freeman, 2nd edition, 1981

Drugs

Breckon, W., *Your Everyday Drugs*, BBC Publications, 1978
Parish, P., *Medicines: A guide for everyone*, Penguin, 5th edition, 1984

Enzymes and hormones

Brush, M., *Understanding Premenstrual Tension*, Pan, 1984
Lewis, J. G., *The Endocrine System*, Churchill Livingstone, 1977
Mason, A. S., *Hormones and The Body*, Penguin, 1976
Palmer, T., *Understanding Enzymes*, Ellis Horwood, 1981

Exercise

Bath, C., *Bodywork*, Foulsham, 1984
Cooper, K., *The Aerobics Way*, Corgi, 1978
Dunne, D., *Yoga Made Easy*, Panther, 1971
Fonda, J., *Jane Fonda's Workout Book*, Allen Lane, 1982
Genova, J., *Work That Body!*, Corgi, 1983

Food and diet

Boycott, R., *The Fastest Diet*, Sphere, 1984
Brown, S., *Sarah Brown's Vegetarian Cookbook*, Dorling Kindersley, 1984
Burkitt, D., *Don't Forget Fibre in Your Diet*, Martin Dunitz, 4th edition, 1983
Cannon, G. and Einzig, H., *Dieting Makes You Fat*, Sphere, 1983
Cott, A., *Fasting: The ultimate diet*, Bantam, 1975
Crystal, D. and Foster, J. L., *Food*, Arnold, 1982
Dutton, D., *Vegetarian Cook Book*, Hamlyn, 1981
Elliot, R., *Gourmet Vegetarian Cooking*, Collins, 1982; Fontana, 1983
Eyton, A., *F-Plan Diet*, Penguin, 1982
Findlater, E., *Wholefood Cooking*, Frederick Muller, 1983
Forsythe, E., *The High-fibre Gourmet*, Pelham, 1983
Highton, N. B. and Highton, R. B., *Home Book of Vegetarian Cooking*, Faber, 2nd edition, 1979
Holme, R., *Pregnancy and Diet*, Penguin, 1985
Horsley, J., *Sugar-free Cookbook*, Prism Press, 1983
Hunt, J. (ed.), *The Very Best of Vegetarian Cooking*, Thorsons, 1984

McLaren, D., *Body Tone Maintenance*, Penguin, 1984
McWilliams, M., *Food Fundamentals*, Wiley, 3rd edition, 1979
Maryon-Davis, A. and Thomas, J., *Diet 2000*, Pan, 1984
Mazel, J., *The Beverly Hills Diet*, Arrow, 1982
        The Beverly Hills Lifetime Diet Plan, Arrow, 1983
Pleshette, J., *Health on your Plate*, Hamlyn, 1983
Tarnower, H. and Baker, S. S., *The Complete Scarsdale Medical Diet*, Bantam, 1980
Walker, C. and Cannon, G., *The Food Scandal*, Century, 1984

Health

Bampfylde, H., *Countdown to a Healthy Baby*, Collins, 1984
        Look Great, Feel Good!, Collins, 1984
Holme, R., *Pregnancy and Diet*, Penguin, 1985
Kenton, L., *The Joy of Beauty*, Century, 1983
Llewellyn Jones, D., *Everywoman: A gynaecological guide for life*, Faber & Faber, 3rd edition, 1982
Lock, S. and Smith, T., *The Medical Risks of Life*, Pelican, 1976

Herbalism

Flüch, H., *Medicinal Plants*, Foulsham, 1976
Lewis, W. H. and Elvin-Lewis, M. P. F., *Medical Botany*, Wiley, 1977
Messegue, M., *Health Secrets of Plants and Herbs*, Collins, 1979; Pan, 1981
Schauenberg, P. and Paris, F., *Guide to Medicinal Plants*, Lutterworth Press, 1977

Homeopathy

Blackie, M. G., *The Patient Not The Cure: The challenge of homeopathy*, Macdonald and Jane's, 1976
Clover, A., *Homeopathy*, Thorsons, 1984
Mitchell, G. R., *Homeopathy*, W. H. Allen, 1975
Vitkoulkas, G., *The Science of Homeopathy*, Grove Press, 1980
        Homeopathy: Medicine of the new man, Thorsons, 1985

Naturopathy

Coleman, V., *Bodypower*, Thames and Hudson, 1984
Mellor, C., *Guide to Natural Health*, Mayflower, 1978
Turner, R. N., *Naturopathic Medicine*, Thorsons, 1984

Negative ion therapy

Soyka, F., *The Ion Effect*, Bantam, 1977

Nutrition
Freedland, R. A. and Briggs, S., *A Biochemical Approach to Nutrition*, Chapman & Hall, 1977
Hunt, S. M., Holbrook, J. M. and Groff, J. L., *Nutrition: Principles and clinical practice*, Wiley, 1980
Ministry of Agriculture, Fisheries and Food, *Manual of Nutrition*, HMSO, 1976
Wilson, E. D., Fisher, K. H. and Garcia, P. A., *Principles of Nutrition*, Wiley, 4th edition, 1979

Sex
Comfort, A. (ed.), *The Joy of Sex*, Quartet, 1974
Rosenberg, J. L., *Total Orgasm*, Wildwood House, 1974

Sleep and stress
Ellis, K., *How To Cope With Insomnia*, Futura, 1984
Lawson, A., *Freedom From Stress*, Thorsons, 1978
Mellor, I., *Sleep*, W. H. Allen, 1981
Oswald, I. and Adam, K., *Insomnia*, Martin Dunitz, 1982
Get a Better Night's Sleep, Martin Dunitz, 1983

Vitamins and minerals
Gildroy, A., *Vitamins and Your Health*, Allen & Unwin, 1982
Hunter, C., *Vitamins: What they are and why we need them*, Thorsons, 1978
Lewin, S., *Vitamin C: Its molecular biology and medical potential*, Academic Press, 1976
Mervyn, L., *Minerals and Your Health*, Unwin, 1980
The Vitamins Explained Simply, Thorsons, 7th edition, 1984
Mindell, E., *The Vitamin Bible*, Arlington Press, 1982
Pauling, L., *Vitamin C, the Common Cold and the Flu*, W. H. Freeman, 2nd edition, 1976
Polunin, M., *Minerals: What they are and why we need them*, Thorsons, 1979

INDEX